Etsuro Mazabei

normal and disturbed MOTILITY OF THE GASTROINTESTINAL TRACT

A.J.P.M. Smout, MD

Department of Gastroenterology, University Hospital of Utrecht
The Netherlands

L.M.A. Akkermans, PhD

Department of Surgery, University Hospital of Utrecht
The Netherlands

WRIGHTSON BIOMEDICAL PUBLISHING LTD
Petersfield

2

Copyright © 1992 by Wrightson Biomedical Publishing Ltd

Reprinted 1994

Editorial Office:

Wrightson Biomedical Publishing Ltd
Ash Barn House, Winchester Road, Stroud,
Petersfield, Hampshire GU32 3PN, UK
Telephone: 0730 265647
Fax: 0730 260368

British Library Cataloguing in Publication Data
A catalogue record for this book is available from the British Library.

ISBN 1 871816 15 7

Composition by Selwood Systems, Midsomer Norton.
Printed in Great Britain by Butler & Tanner Ltd, Frome.

Contents

Abbreviations

5-HT	=	5-hydroxytryptamine (i.e. serotonin)
ACh	=	acetylcholine
ATP	=	adenosine triphosphate
ATPase	=	enzyme that splits ATP
CCK	=	cholecystokinin
CCK8	=	8-peptide of cholecystokinin
CIIP	=	chronic idiopathic intestinal pseudo-obstruction
CIP	=	chronic intestinal pseudo-obstruction
CVA	=	cerebrovascular accident
EAS	=	external anal sphincter
ECA	=	electrical control activity
EGG	=	electrogastrography
EMG	=	electromyography
ENS	=	enteric nervous system
ERA	=	electrical response activity
ERCP	=	endoscopic retrograde cholangiopancreaticography
HIDA	=	hepatobiliary IDA
HSV	=	highly selective vagotomy
IAS	=	internal anal sphincter
IBD	=	inflammatory bowel disease
IDA	=	iminodiacetic acid
LOS	=	lower oesophageal sphincter
MMC	=	(interdigestive) migrating motor complex
UOS	=	upper oesophageal sphincter
VIP	=	vasoactive intestinal polypeptide

Foreword

In recent years some major discoveries
have been made about the motility of
the gastrointestinal tract and its
dysfunction. Moreover, the range of
therapeutic options for these disorders
has expanded considerably. There is a
great need for a practical overview of
these developments with the accent on
motility disturbances and their treatment.
This book is intended as both a
handbook and a reference book. It is as
practical as possible, with advice for
treatment and overviews of diagnoses.
We hope that it will be useful in the
clinical practice of both general
practitioner and specialist. Comments
and criticisms are most welcome.

Many persons have contributed to the
realization of this book. In particular we
wish to thank Paul van Dongen, PhD, for
his unflagging effort and enthusiasm.

André J.P.M. Smout
Louis M.A. Akkermans

6

Introduction

Gastroenterology has witnessed a revolution in the past 20 years. In addition to radiology and rigid endoscopy, flexible endoscopy, manometry, pH-monitoring and scintigraphy have become available. As a consequence, many more disorders of the gastrointestinal tract can be identified. Also, more effective and more selective drugs and new and refined surgical techniques have been developed.

Structures and functions of the digestive tract

In the past few decades our knowledge of the normal structure and function of the digestive tract has substantially expanded.

◆ For 25 years, it has been possible to identify neurotransmitters, hormones and peptides in specific types of cells. In the past 10 years in particular these techniques have been considerably improved. As a result, our knowledge of what neurotransmitters and biologically active substances are present in the gastrointestinal tract has grown enormously.

◆ Researchers now have recourse to selective agonists and antagonists of a large number of receptors. These are powerful tools, not only for studying and locating various receptors, but also for determining the effect of specific biologically active substances on the gastrointestinal tract.

◆ We now know much more about the normal functioning of the gastrointestinal tract. We have methods for prolonged data recording in the gastrointestinal tract of healthy persons (and patients). Normal motility, from the oesophagus to the anus, can now be investigated more intensively.

Diagnosis

Older readers will recall that diagnostic methods were once confined to a detailed history-taking, auscultation and X-ray and blood examination. This circumstance of course limited the number of disorders that could be reliably identified. There was a large category of patients whose abdominal disorders were not understood. For lack of a better explanation, some doctors interpreted these complaints as mainly psychogenic. Since that time we have learned that many symptoms are in fact associated with motility disturbances of the digestive tract. Only with the development of new investigational techniques has it been possible to identify these disturbances. Some of them are secondary to other disorders. Consequently and naturally enough, diagnoses have become much more precise. This book gives an overview of the present state of the art.

Treatment

A survey of older pharmacology handbooks on the drug therapy of stomach and intestinal disorders will convince you of the progress that has been made in this field. In 1969 the most important groups of drugs were laxatives and antacids, whilst acids (now obsolete) and adsorbents were also still used. In addition, anthelmintics were also cited (Kuschinsky and Lüllmann 1969). Ten years later the arrival of prokinetics, H_2-blockers and selective antidiarrhoeals was announced. Today there are new prokinetics and drugs that inhibit gastric acid secretion. Along with antidiarrhoeals and laxatives, this is the most important group of drugs in the treatment of motility disorders of the gastrointestinal tract. Thanks to the new diagnostic methods, treatment can be better tailored to the patient.

Reference

Kuschinsky G, Lüllmann H. Kurzes Lehrbuch der Pharmacologie, 4de druk. Stuttgart: Georg Thieme, 1969

Anatomy and physiology

Anatomy of the gastrointestinal tract

The digestive tract is a hollow tube consisting of separate compartments. Each of these compartments has its own structure, which in turn corresponds to a particular function.

Introduction

The gastrointestinal tract can simplistically be described as a hollow tube, extending from the mouth to the anus. The diameter of this tube is not the same throughout its length: there are widenings and narrowings, so that the gastrointestinal tract can be divided into the following compartments: oesophagus, stomach, small intestine, large intestine, rectum and anus: Some compartments are separated from one another by sphincters, which, when appropriate, open and close, thereby sending the food (whether or not digested), in appropriate quantities, in the right direction. Also the wall of the tube varies with the compartment. The basic structure of the gastrointestinal tact is the same throughout its length, however. The differences between compartments are nothing more than variations on the theme of the basic structure. Owing to these variations, each part performs a characteristic function.

Intermezzo 1
Specializations in food absorption

In order that nutrients should be absorbed and waste excreted, the internal milieu must be brought into contact with the external milieu. In single-celled organisms this contact is achieved rather simply: they lie with the thin cell membrane directly facing the external milieu. The larger the organism, the greater the number of cells and the more specialized the cells become. Not every cell in such organisms borders on the outside. A need thus arises for transport from cell to cell. With increasing growth and specialization comes the capacity for transient food storage and processing of large food particles into substances that can be absorbed by the cell. Physical and chemical fragmentation and dissolution (i.e. "digestion") must be adapted to the nature and quantity of the food ingested by the organism. Transport within the body has thus become essential for efficient processing and absorption. Specializations then develop these functions:
— transport and processing in the external milieu (the gastrointestinal tract)
— absorption from the external milieu (transport systems in the intestinal wall)
— transport in the internal milieu (heart and blood vessels).

The basic structure

The basic structure consists of a number of layers (Figure 1). From the lumen outwards, these are as follows: the mucosa, the submucosa, the muscularis and the serosa.

◆ The **mucosa** separates the external milieu from the internal compartment. There are also glandular cells in the mucosa.

◆ The **submucosa** consists primarily of collagen and elastic fibres. In this layer is situated, amongst other elements, a network of nerves, Meissner's plexus, or the submucosal plexus.

◆ Under the submucosa lies the **muscularis**, which consists of two muscular coats: an inner layer of circular muscle, and surrounding it, a layer of longitudinal muscle. This nerve plexus plays an important role in the motility of the gastrointestinal tract.

◆ The **outer layer** of the gastrointestinal tract consists mainly of connective tissue and elastic fibres. In the stomach and intestines, these constitute the peritoneum, or serosa. In it pass blood vessels, lymph vessels and nerve fibres. As for the oesophagus, the outer layer is an elastic, non-serous membrane.

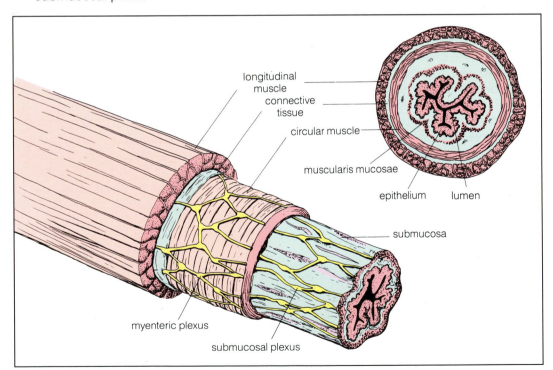

longitudinal muscle
connective tissue
circular muscle
muscularis mucosae
epithelium
lumen
submucosa
myenteric plexus
submucosal plexus

Figure 1: The basic structure of the digestive tract, showing the various layers of the oesophagus.

The oesophagus

The oesophagus is a tube about 20 cm long, delimited by two sphincters: the upper oesophageal sphincter and the lower oesophageal sphincter.

Mucosa
The coating of the oesophagus consists of a multi-layered mucous squamous cell epithelium. A mono-layered cylindrical epithelium can be found only in the distal centimetres. The transition zone between the two types of epithelium is abrupt and runs zigzag, and is for this reason also called the Z-line. In the mucosa there are two types of mucous glands: the cardia glands and the oesophageal glands. The latter extend into the submucosa.

Submucosa
In the oesophagus the oesophageal glands extend to the submucosa. Ganglia are scarce in the submucosal plexus. However, there are many nerve fibres that approach the border of the epithelium.

Muscular layer
The oesophagus is delimited on the upper and lower end by a sphincter: the upper oesophageal sphincter (UOS) and the lower oesophageal sphincter (LOS).

◆ The **UOS** is formed by the musculus cricopharyngeus, which is loop-shaped and attached to the cricoid. This is the most distal part of the interior pharyngeal constrictor.
◆ The circular muscle of the **oesophagus** connects with the UOS. The longitudinal muscle is also attached to the cricoid. In the muscularis of the oesophagus there are two types of muscle tissue: striated and smooth muscle. Roughly speaking, the upper third of the oesophagus consists of striated muscle, the middle third of striated and smooth muscle and the lower third of smooth muscle. The myenteric plexus contains relatively few ganglia. The bundles extend mainly abroad, with thinner connections that extend laterally.
◆ The **LOS** is not a real anatomical sphincter. Rather it is a physiological sphincter, whilst the wall in this part of the oesophagus is somewhat asymmetrically thickened.

The external elastic layer
The external layer of the oesophagus contains relatively numerous fibres. In this fashion the oesophagus can be transiently stretched by a passing food particle and the food passes smoothly. In the connective tissue are found mainly blood vessels and nerve fibre branches. The vagus nerve forms a rough network in this layer.

The stomach

The stomach is a pouch-shaped organ that is delimited on the upper surface by the LOS and on the lower surface by the pylorus. The most important parts of this organ are, from the proximal to the distal end: the fundus, the corpus and the antrum (Figure 2).

Mucosa

Whereas the upper surface of the mucosa of the oesophagus is smooth, that of the stomach is convoluted, especially in the corpus. As a result of this enlargement of the upper surface area, the contents of the stomach are thoroughly exposed there to the stomach wall. In the stomach there is a single layer of highly cylindrical epithelium. Throughout the stomach this epithelium contains mucous cells that produce a mucous layer that protects the stomach against excoriation by acid and pepsin. In the corpus there are mucous tubules with mucous cells, parietal cells and chief cells. The parietal cells produce hydrochloric acid and intrinsic factor. The chief cells produce pepsinogen. The glandular tubules terminate in microscopic pits called foveolae. In addition, the epithelial cells have microvilli. The epithelium of the stomach is marked by a high turnover, the life of the epithelial cells being only 2–4 days.

Submucosa

Just as in the oesophagus, the submucosal plexus in the stomach contains few ganglia. The submucosal plexus of the stomach is not continuous with that of small intestine but is interrupted in the pylorus area.

Muscular layer

The muscular coat of the stomach differs from that of the oesophagus and the intestines. In the proximal part of the stomach there is an inner additional coat of oblique muscle. Wrapped around this are the circular and longitudinal muscles. The thickness of the muscular coat increases distally, reaching a maximum in the pylorus. The myenteric plexus extends from the oesophagus to the stomach without interruption. In the fundus the plexus still contains few ganglia, but in the antrum and pylorus the number and size of the ganglia increase sharply. The muscular coats of the pylorus and duodenum are separated from one another by a septum consisting of connective tissue. The myenteric plexus of the stomach is continuous with that of the pylorus and the small intestine. This structural aspect plays an important role in the co-ordination of gastroduodenal contractions (antroduodenal co-ordination, p. 95).

Serosa

The serosa of the stomach connects with the greater and lesser omentum on the surfaces of greater and of lesser curvature. Numerous blood vessels and nerve fibre branches pervade the serosa.

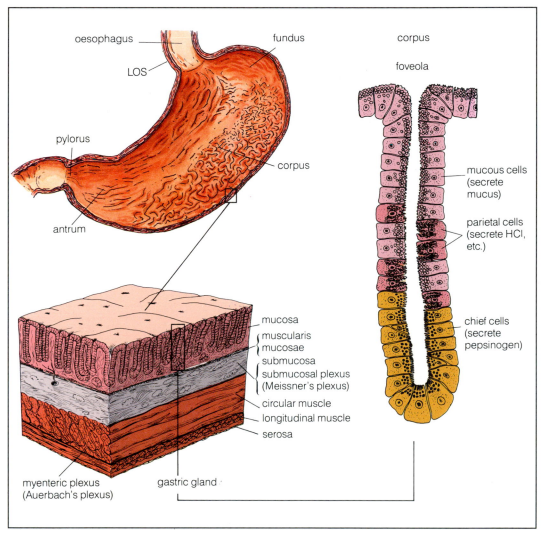

oesophagus

fundus

corpus

LOS

foveola

pylorus

corpus

antrum

mucous cells
(secrete
mucus)

parietal cells
(secrete HCl,
etc.)

mucosa

muscularis
mucosae
submucosa
submucosal plexus
(Meissner's plexus)

circular muscle

longitudinal muscle

serosa

chief cells
(secrete
pepsinogen)

myenteric plexus
(Auerbach's plexus)

gastric gland

Figure 2: Structure of the wall of the stomach with a schematic drawing of the glandular layer of the corpus and antrum.

The gallbladder and bile ducts

The liver contains smaller bile ducts that unite to form larger ducts, and ultimately the left and right hepatic duct (Figure 3). These unite to form the common bile duct. About 3 cm downstream the cystic duct (which serves as a passageway to and from the gallbladder) empties into the common bile duct. From this point on, the passage in question is referred to as the choledochus (common bile duct), which, after about 7.5 cm empties into the papilla of Vater in the duodenum. Generally the duct leaving the pancreas (the pancreatic duct) also ends in this papilla. The gallbladder is a pear-shaped organ 7–10 cm long and 3 cm wide (maximum). The transport of the bile to and from the gallbladder takes place in the same duct, the cystic duct, which is 3–4 cm long.

Mucosa
The gallbladder and bile ducts are coated by a single layer of cylindrical epithelium. This membrane contains mucous glands and these are particularly numerous in the bile ducts. In the gallbladder the epithelium carries out active resorption of water.

Submucosa
In the bile ducts there is no submucosal plexus in the strict sense of the term. In the gallbladder, however, there is a well-defined submucosal plexus.

The muscular layer
In the large bile ducts the muscular layer is almost absent. The layer between the submucosa and the serosa consists of

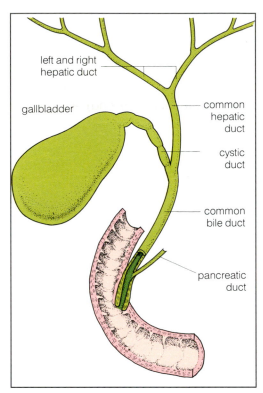

Figure 3: The macroscopic structure of the gallbladder and the major bile ducts.

connective tissue, smooth muscle fibres being few and far between. It is only at the extremity of the common bile duct that a greater quantity of smooth muscle tissue is to be found, which forms the sphincter of Oddi. There is considerable muscle tissue in the wall of the gallbladder, although one cannot speak of a distinct layer of longitudinal and circular muscle. Longitudinal muscle is abundant and circular muscle scarce.

Serosa
It is via the serosa that blood vessels and nerve fibre branches reach the bile ducts and gallbladder.

The small intestine

The small intestine is a long twisting tube about 5 m long. It consists of a short duodenum (about 25 cm long), a jejunum (about 2 m long) and an ileum (about 3 m long).

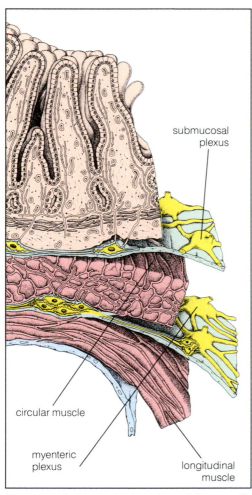

Figure 4: Schematic drawing of the small intestine, peeled apart to show the positions of the muscle layers and nerves.

Mucosa
In the small intestine the surface is much more marked by folds than in the stomach. There are microscopic folds, numerous villi and microvilli (Figure 4). It is for this reason that the surface area is more than 500 times greater than that of a hollow tube. The mucous membrane of the small intestine has about the same area as a football field. The glandular epithelium consists of a single layer. Just as in the stomach, it has a short life and after a few days is replaced by new cells, which push to the top from the base of the villi. Between the epithelial cells, which carry out water resorption, goblet cells are found. This structure characterizes the entire small intestine.

Submucosa
The small intestine houses a highly developed submucosal plexus with numerous ganglia. Two layers can be distinguished in this plexus: one internal and the other external.

Muscular layer
A regular structure consisting of circular and longitudinal muscle is also found in the small intestine. The muscularis is thinner here than in the distal part of the stomach. The myenteric plexus is highly developed here and contains numerous and large ganglia.

Serosa
The serosa is threaded by blood vessels and nerve tracts that pass to and from the small intestine. The serosa of the small intestine connects with the mesenterium. The position of the small intestine is highly variable. At the level of the duodenum and the ileocaecal juncture the position is fixed.

The large intestine

The large intestine is about 1.5 m long. From its proximal to its distal end, it consists of the following parts: caecum, ascending colon, transverse colon, descending colon, sigmoid colon and rectum.

Mucosa

The wall of the large intestine has a fairly smooth surface without folds. The epithelium consists of a single layer of tall cylindrical cells, with more goblet cells than in the small intestine. Furthermore, there is some enlargement of the surface due to the formation of crypts. Distally in the rectum there are longitudinal folds, whilst the crypts become shallower and disappear. On the other hand, there are circular folds in the form of haustra. These are not anatomical constrictions but contractions of the smooth circular muscle. They give the large intestine its characteristic macroscopic appearance. Immediately above the anus there is an abrupt transition to multi-layered squamous cell epithelium, which at the external sphincter becomes the epithelium of the skin.

Submucosa

In the colon the thickness of the submucosal plexus again diminishes. Here too are found an internal plexus and an external plexus. In addition there is a third, more outward-lying layer (the extreme external plexus). The sub-mucosa of the large intestine consists largely of lymphatic tissue, which serves as an additional protective layer.

Muscular layer

In the colon the inner layer of the circular muscle has the same structure as the other compartments. The outer muscular layer here, however, is different: the longitudinal muscle in the wall of the colon consists of three bands. Between these bands there is hardly any longitudinal muscle. In the rectosigmoid the bundles give way to the longitudinal muscle of the rectum. The structure of the myenteric plexus in the colon is comparable to that in the small intestine. The number of ganglia gradually declines distally.

Serosa

The ascending colon and transverse colon do not have a mesenterium. In contrast the descending colon and sigmoid colon have a mesenterium and are therefore rather mobile.

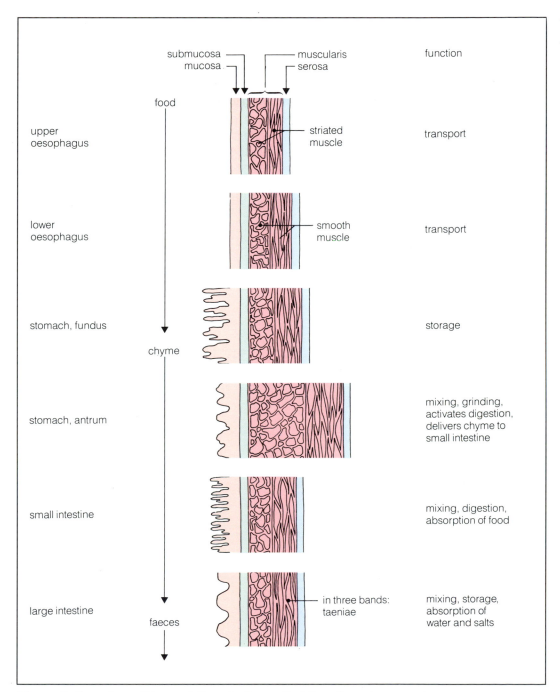

Figure 5: Overview of the variations in the wall of the alimentary canal.

The rectum

The rectum is the continuation of the large intestine. In the rectum there is a distinct enteric nervous system with a myenteric plexus and submucosa. Whilst the large intestine is traversed by three distinct bands (taeniae) of longitudinal muscle, in the rectum these bands unite to form a continuous layer that extends around its entire circumference.

The anal canal

The distal extremity of the rectum is characterized by a narrowing. The juncture between the rectum and the anus is located here. The action of the anus is determined by smooth and striated muscle. Muscles of the pelvic floor also play a role. The structure of the anal region is so distinct that it is dealt with separately in Chapter 11 (p. 172).

Innervation of the gastrointestinal tract

The movements of the stomach and intestines are primarily under the control of the autonomic nervous system. In addition, the gut wall has its own nervous system, the enteric nervous system (ENS). It was once believed that this was a simple relay system of the autonomic nervous system. It is now known that the ENS co-ordinates and integrates the activities of the stomach and intestines.

26

Introduction

Almost all the activity of the digestive system takes place outside our control and without our perceiving it. Only at the beginning and at the end of the gastrointestinal tract can we consciously influence its movements. In particular, striated (voluntary) muscle is found at the proximal end of the oesophagus and the anus (Figure 6). Swallowing and defaecation (or retention) can be consciously influenced. The other activities of the stomach and intestines proceed automatically; they are controlled by the sympathetic and the parasympathetic nervous system and by a network of nerve cells in the gut wall called the enteric nervous system (ENS).

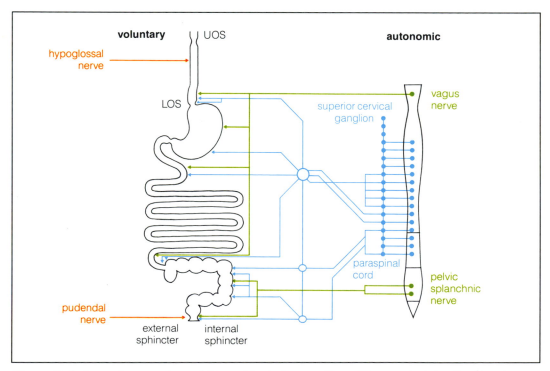

Figure 6: Schematic overview of the extrinsic innervation of the gastrointestinal tract.

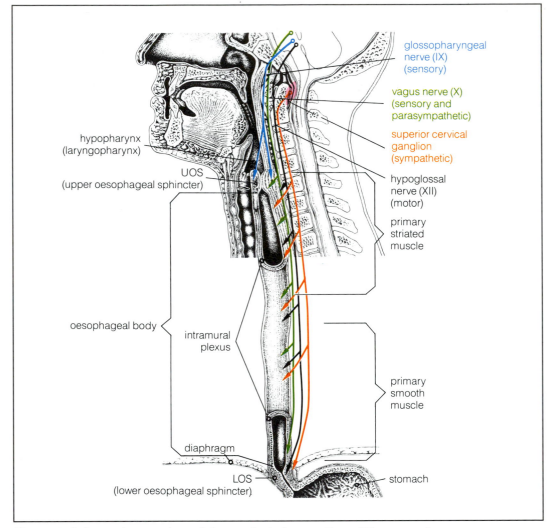

Figure 7: Schematic overview of the extrinsic innervation of the oesophagus.

Extrinsic innervation

The extrinsic nervous system consists principally of an autonomic nervous network, with only a small number of voluntary nerve fibres.

Autonomic innervation

Traditionally the autonomic nervous system is divided into two components: the sympathetic and parasympathetic.

◆ **Parasympathetic** innervation is provided primarily by the vagus nerve, whose cell bodies lie in the brain stem. The vagus nerve leaves the brain and passes to the oesophagus, where it branches into a rough plexus-like structure, which innervates the oesophagus. From here, two bundles pass through the diaphragm, branching off to the stomach, the small intestine and the ascending colon. The vagus nerve does not consist exclusively of (efferent) parasympathetic fibres; a large portion of the fibres of the vagus nerve are (afferent) sensory fibres. These provide the brain with information on the state of the stomach and intestines. The importance of the innervation by the vagus nerve becomes particularly clear after vagotomy. The

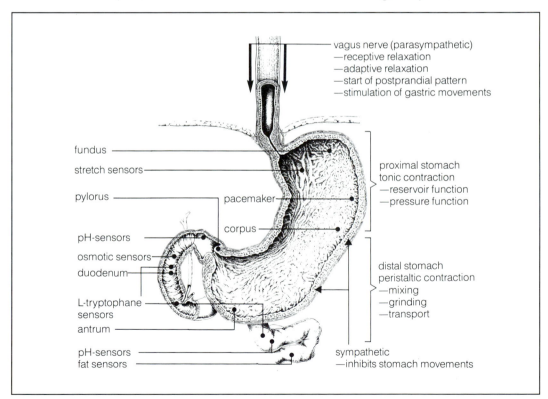

Figure 8: Schematic overview of the extrinsic innervation of the stomach.

movements of the stomach are then impaired or even absent. The distal part of the colon and rectum is parasympathetically innervated by other fibres, in particular the pelvic splanchnic nerves that leave the sacral region of the spinal cord. The parasympathetic fibres pass directly from the central nervous system to the intestine and end in the myenteric plexus and submucosa. The principal neurotransmitter in parasympathetic control is acetylcholine.

◆ **Sympathetic** innervation arises from the thoracolumbar portion of the spinal cord. Branches from this section arrive at the sympathetic ganglia (the coeliac ganglion, amongst others). Here the fibres synapse with the postganglionic nerve cells, whose fibres follow the

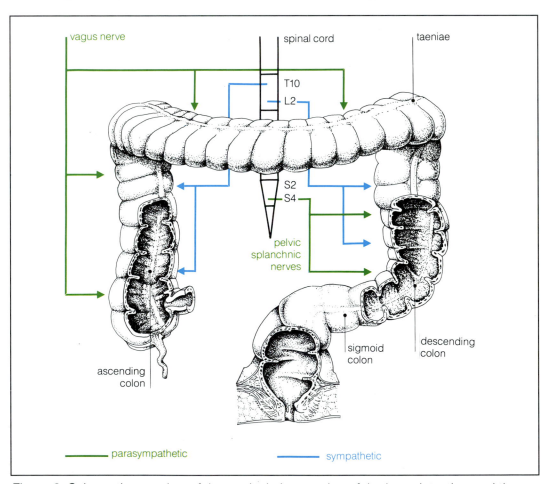

Figure 9: Schematic overview of the extrinsic innervation of the large intestine and the anus.

mesenteric vessels and end in the intramural plexus. The most important neurotransmitter of this system is noradrenalin.

Previously the autonomic nervous system was thought to consist of a sympathetic and parasympathetic division, with noradrenalin and acetylcholine respectively as neurotransmitters. It is now known that there are many other transmitters. Some of these are found together with noradrenalin or acetylcholine in the same nerve fibres (coexistence).

Voluntary influence on the alimentary canal

In the alimentary canal only the mouth, throat and upper oesophageal sphincter at one end and the anus at the other can be voluntarily controlled.

◆ The hypopharynx and the upper oesophageal sphincter contain striated muscle that is innervated by the hypoglossal nerve. In this way voluntary control over swallowing can be exerted.

◆ The external anal sphincter consists of striated muscle that is innervated by the pudendal nerve. These fibres keep the anus constricted except during defaecation.

Intrinsic innervation

The myenteric plexus and submucosa are located in the gut wall and together they form the ENS. The myenteric plexus lies between the circular and the longitudinal muscle whereas the submucosal plexus is situated in the submucosa (Figure 10). Previously the ENS was thought to be a simple relay station in the parasympathetic nervous

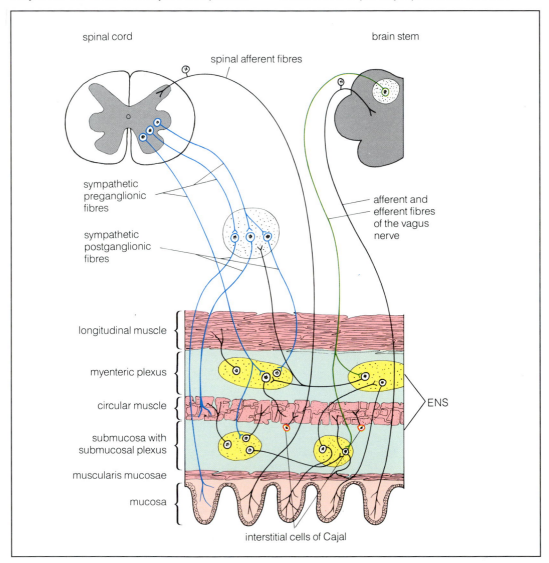

Figure 10: Connections between the extrinsic and the intrinsic nervous network in the gastrointestinal tract.

system in which impulses were conveyed unmodified from pre- to postganglionic end-fibres. The ENS was seen as a simple extension of the vagus nerve. It is now known that the ENS consists of a large number of sensory, integrative and motor neurons. A substantial part of the integration of the gastrointestinal movements occurs in the ENS and it is for this reason that it is referred to as the "little brain of the gut" The ENS comprises a number of networks of ganglia. Between the ganglia is situated a network of nerve fibres called the primary plexus. This element is found throughout the gastrointestinal system. The submucosal plexus houses only the primary plexus. But in the myenteric plexus smaller branches are found that make contact with one another and the resulting entity is called the secondary plexus. Finally an even finer network, the tertiary plexus, can be identified. There are upwards of 10 million nerve cells in the ENS. A broad range of neurotransmitters and hormones has been discovered in connection with the ENS (Intermezzo 2).

The motor end-plate in the striated muscles is often taken as a model of neuromuscular signal transmission. It does not apply to smooth muscle cells however. Motor neurons have axons that extend over greater distances between the muscle fibres. Packets of neurotransmitter are transported by the axons. These appear as thickenings (varicosities) at regular distances from one another. From them, transmitter substance is secreted. The transmitter must bridge a fair distance (about 1 mm) to the receptors on the smooth muscle cells. A nerve cell generally exerts action on several smooth muscle cells.

Oesophagus

The myenteric plexus in the oesophagus contains relatively few ganglia. Generally bundles of thick fibres are found that extend craniocaudally. Long thin axons are found in the longitudinal muscle, whilst in the circular muscle, nerve fibres tend to be more dispersed. The circular muscle fibres are not innervated directly by the nerve fibres but indirectly by interneurons. In the submucosal plexus, fibres are fairly densely concentrated but there are no ganglia. It is possible that these fibres arise from the ganglionic cells in the myenteric plexus.

Stomach

In the myenteric plexus of the fundus there are relatively few ganglia and the secondary and tertiary plexus are not very developed. In the antrum, on the other hand, the ganglia are large and dense and there is a well-developed network. Here the plexus contains the shunt fascicles, which, from the oesophagus, are distributed over the stomach. It is possible that these are vagal nerve fibres that, in addition to directly innervating the stomach, follow another pathway. The submucosal plexus of the stomach contains relatively few ganglionic cells.

Intermezzo 2
Neurotransmitters and hormones

A wide assortment of neurotransmitters and hormones is found in the ENS (Table 1). It was once believed that there was a firm distinction between neurotransmitters and hormones but it is now known that there are many intermediate forms. An umbrella term for neurotransmitter- and hormone-like substances is messengers. These messengers can be secreted in different ways.

◆ **Neurocrine secretion.** The basis of this mechanism is classical synaptic binding. There is point-to-point contact. The synaptic knobs lie right next to the target cell (a synaptic cleft is about 0.03 μm wide, Figure 11). This is the prototypal contact for neurotransmission.

◆ **Paracrine secretion.** Cells secrete substances that influence locally an area of only a few square millimetres. These cells can be actual neurons with dendrites and an excitable axon; often this axon has varicosities from which the messengers are released. Cells that bear no morphological resemblance to neurons also contribute to paracrine secretion.

◆ **Endocrine secretion.** This mechanism involves actual hormones. Cells secrete substances into the blood. These substances are capable of affecting tissues and organs located throughout the body.

In the ENS the same messengers are found as in the brain. Also in the brain there is paracrine secretion of a variety of messengers. In many cases several messengers are found in the same neuron. A number of messengers are known to stimulate or inhibit movement (Table 1). We hope that detailed information in this connection will be forthcoming in the near future. It is well known that different types of motility occur in the gastrointestinal tract, for example phasic contractions and tonal contractions (whether or not attended by action potentials). These lead to integrated motility patterns like peristaltic, haustral and mass contractions, which can be integrated with a postprandial or an interdigestive pattern. We should very much like to know how each messenger contributes to the different motility patterns. This knowledge is also important in drug therapy; it is evident that by stimulating or blocking the receptors for these messengers one can affect the movements of the stomach and intestines in many different ways. When we have a more detailed knowledge of the action of the different messengers, we shall perhaps be able to exert a much more selective and better directed control over the gastrointestinal tract.

stimulating	inhibiting
– acetylcholine (ACh)	– dopamine (DA)
– serotonin (5-hydroxytryptamine)	– noradrenalin (NA)
– histamine	– glucagon
– cholecystokinin (CCK)	– vasoactive intestinal poly-
– angiotensin (ANG)	peptide (VIP)
– motilin	– somatostatin
– gastrin	– enkephalin (ENK)

Table 1. Effect of a number of messengers on the motility of the stomach and intestines.

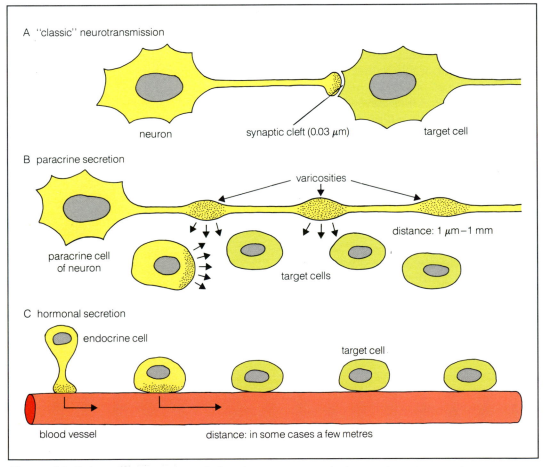

Figure 11: Schematic overview of classic neurotransmission and endocrine (hormonal) and paracrine secretion.

The gallbladder and the bile ducts

The gallbladder and bile ducts are parasympathetically innervated by a branch of the vagus nerve. The sympathetic fibres reach this organ from the coeliac ganglion. In the wall of the gallbladder itself there are a mucosal and a myenteric plexus. In the wall of the bile ducts, although there are nerve cells, these are not clustered in a well-defined intramural plexus. On the other hand in the sphincter of Oddi there is a dense network of nerve cells.

The small intestine

The myenteric plexus of the small intestine is comparable to that of the antrum; it houses numerous ganglia and a dense network. A well-developed secondary and tertiary plexus can also be found here. The structure is about the same throughout the small intestine. The submucosal plexus is very elaborate in the small intestine, to the point where two layers can be identified: a network directly under the muscularis mucosae (Meissner's plexus in the narrow sense of the term), and a network next to circular muscle. The two layers are connected to one another. In addition to the myenteric plexus and the submucosal plexus a few smaller nervous networks are located in the small intestine. These lie in the serosa, between the circular muscle and the lamina propria, and do not contain any ganglia.

The large intestine

The myenteric plexus of the colon is similar to that of the small intestine. The ganglia become narrower aborad. The rectum houses few ganglia. The secondary and the tertiary networks found there are not very elaborate. In the distal colon shunt fascicles are found that arise from the pelvic plexus. Exactly as in the oesophagus, these form a kind of expressway; together, they ensure a well-coordinated transit of the faeces. The submucosal plexus of the large intestine also consists of two layers but is not as dense as that of the small intestine.

Conclusion: the ENS and autonomic innervation

In some of the functions of the stomach and intestines the ENS is more important than the autonomic nervous network. An isolated stomach and isolated parts of the intestine can effect peristaltic contractions owing to the ENS. In fasting subjects the gastrointestinal tract displays a complex gastric motility and secretion pattern known as the migrating motor complex (MMC, p. 47). It is assumed that this cycle of activity is primarily controlled by the ENS. We shall later see that gastric emptying is jointly determined by the amount and composition of the food (p. 98). This information is registered by mechano-, chemo- and osmo-receptors. On the basis of this input the movements of the stomach and intestines are controlled (by the vagus nerve and the ENS). For other aspects of gastrointestinal function, autonomic innervation is more important. The sight or chewing of food (or even the expectation of food) acts as a stimulus, so that the vagus nerve stimulates gastric acid production in the first phase of this secretion. Immediately after a swallowing movement the proximal stomach relaxes for about 20 seconds under the action of the vagus nerve. This phase is known as receptive relaxation (p. 90). When the stomach is stretched by food, receptive relaxation gives way to longer-lasting relaxation (adaptive relaxation, p. 90) of the smooth muscle of the stomach, effected by sensory and motor fibres of the vagus nerve. The vagus nerve also plays a part in activating the special gastric motility pattern of the stomach and intestines after a meal, i.e. the postprandial pattern. And lastly, the vagus in general stimulates the motility of stomach and intestines. The sympathetic fibres have an antagonistic action. When sympathetic fibres are stimulated, the motility of stomach and intestines is inhibited.

Basic physiology

The movements of the gastrointestinal tract are brought about by the smooth muscle cells. In this chapter we shall explain how the activity of these cells arises. We shall then give an overview of the movements of the gastrointestinal tract after a meal and between meals.

Introduction

In the investigation of the physiology of the gastrointestinal tract, attention is initially focused primarily on the secretion of digestive juices, which convert food into nutrient substances that can be absorbed. At least as important for adequate functioning of the gastrointestinal tract are the following processes: mixing, grinding and transporting. For optimal activity the movements of the separate parts of the gastrointestinal tract must be adjusted to one another and to the food bolus. Nerve cells inside and outside the gastrointestinal tract co-ordinate these movements and secretion.

Intermezzo 3
Digestion in compartments

Food cannot be absorbed by the body in its initial state. The organic nutrients must first be reduced by enzymes to substances that are suitable for resorption. The gut wall also consists of such organic components. Thus in principle the gut wall is also liable to digestion by digestive enzymes. Fortunately our bodies can avoid such action. Important in this connection is the fact that the gastrointestinal tract consists of compartments, which are more or less separate from one another. Each compartment makes its own contribution to digestion, secreting its own enzymes. The mucous membrane of each compartment is protected against its own enzymes but not against those of other compartments. The different enzymes in the different compartments are successively released on the food. In this manner the gut wall is never exposed to all enzymes at the same time. The stomach contains the proteolytic enzyme pepsin, which is optimally effective in an acidic milieu. If pepsin comes into contact with (half-digested) food in the duodenum, it is inactivated there since the milieu is alkaline. In the duodenum the proteolytic enzyme trypsin is secreted and is therefore optimally effective. In contrast, trypsin is inactivated in the acidic milieu of the stomach if it ends up there as a result of reflux. The compartments are separated from one another by sphincters. Through the movements of the oesophagus, stomach and intestines the food is transported from one compartment to another.

Action of the smooth muscle cells

The smooth muscle cells induce the contractions of the stomach and intestines. Two types of contraction are distinguished:
— short, (more or less) rhythmic, **phasic**
— long, **tonic**
In the proximal stomach, the gallbladder and the sphincters tonic contractions predominate; in the distal stomach and the small intestine phasic contractions do so.

The electrical control activity

Just as in all body cells the smooth muscle cells of the stomach and intestines are negatively charged inside; there is a potential difference across the membrane. This difference is not constant but fluctuates more or less rhythmically (Figure 12A). At the point at which the greatest potential difference is reached the cell depolarizes and remains depolarized for 3 to 10 seconds. After this interval the cell repolarizes. The up- and downswings continue unabated, whether the cell

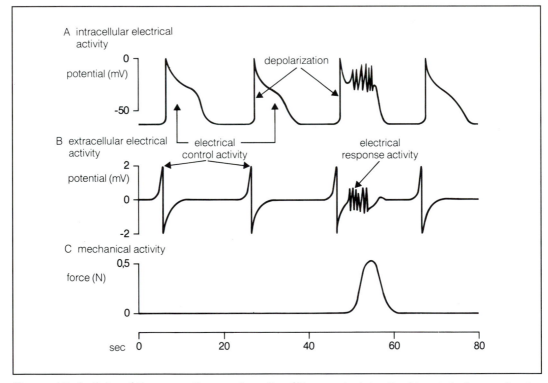

Figure 12: Activity of the smooth muscle cells of the gastrointestinal tract during a phasic contraction. A: Intracellular signal: rhythmic fluctuations of the membrane potential with or without action potentials. B: Extracellular signal measured with an electrode in the muscle. C: The force delivered by the muscle. (It should be noted that the muscle contracts only during action potentials.)

contracts concurrently or not. This pattern is known as the electrical control activity (ECA). The frequency of the electrical control activity is 3 cycles per minute in the stomach. These potential fluctuations can also be registered with extracellular electrodes (Figure 12B), and even with electrodes on the skin (electrogastrography, Figure 134, p. 294). The highest frequency of the electrical control activity in the small bowel is found in the duodenum (about 12 cycles per minute) and the lowest in the terminal ileum (8–9 cycles per minute). The electrical control activity arises in the pacemaker regions. In the stomach the pacemaker lies on the greater curvature and in the small intestine pacemakers are distributed over the duodenum. Previously physiologists thought that the pacemaker rhythm was evoked by smooth muscle cells themselves. Now there is strong evidence that the interstitial cells of Cajal (a specialized type of nerve cell, Figure 10, p. 32) generate the rhythm; exactly how these cells perform this function is not yet known. The interstitial cells of Cajal transmit the rhythm to the smooth muscle cells. Every wave of this rhythmic activity is propagated distally at a speed of between 0.5 and 4 cm/s. The waves proceed distally whether or not there are concurrent contractions.

Phasic contractions: action potentials

In the depolarized state the smooth muscle cells can suddenly display one or more action (spike) potentials (Figure 12). These spike potentials are always attended by a muscle contraction and the production of these potentials is called the electrical response activity (ERA). These phasic contractions occur when the smooth muscle cells are stimulated during the appropriate phase of the electrical control activity. Consequently the electrical control activity determines the times at which phasic contractions can arise and the direction in which they can be propagated. Since the electrical control activity is propagated distally, the phasic contractions proceed distally also.

From depolarization to contraction

Why is it that some depolarizations cause smooth muscle cells to contract and others do not? The outcome is determined by motorneurons of the myenteric plexus. These motorneurons innervate the smooth muscle cells. When the motorneurons produce action potentials, acetylcholine is liberated. Acetylcholine stimulates the muscarinic receptors on the smooth muscle cells, causing an influx of calcium ions into the smooth muscle cells, which in turn brings about a contraction. The motorneurons that produce this chain of events belong to the ENS. They are affected by other neurons of the ENS, by mechano- and chemosensors of the stomach and intestines, and by the sympathetic and parasympathetic nervous systems.

Peristaltic contractions

Peristaltic contractions are phasic contractions of the circular muscle that are propagated a certain distance aborally*. Of crucial importance to the production of peristalsis is the electrical control activity. But the neurons of the ENS also play their part. A particular form of peristaltic contraction is the peristaltic reflex. This is induced by a stimulus from the intestines (e.g. a food bolus). This stimulus elicits the following movements (Figure 13).

◆ The segment of the stomach or intestine proximal to the bolus contracts. At the same time the circular muscle contracts and the longitudinal muscle relaxes.
◆ Simultaneously the distal segment prepares to receive the bolus: the circular muscle in this segment relaxes and the longitudinal muscle contracts.

This contraction wave is slowly conducted distally. The ENS neurons ensure that the contraction–relaxation pattern proceeds smoothly.

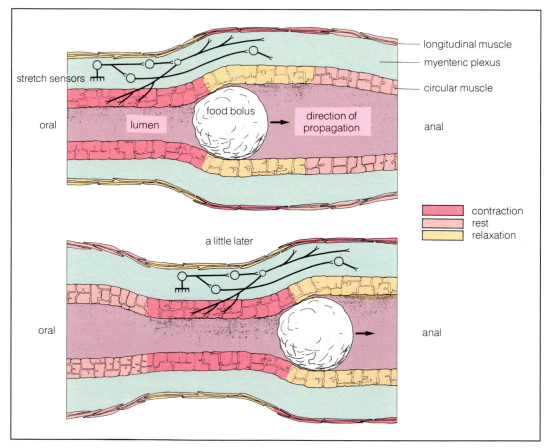

Figure 13: A peristaltic contraction wave is propagated through a segment of the intestine.

*Formerly it was believed that all movements of the stomach and intestines were peristaltic contractions. Thus the word "peristaltic" was erroneously used to refer to every movement of these organs.

Tonic contractions

In principle tonic contractions occur throughout the gastrointestinal tract. However, they are prominent in the proximal stomach, the gallbladder and all the sphincters. There are two forms of tonic contractions (Figure 14):

◆ Tonic contractions without action potentials (spike-free). In the smooth muscle cells that produce this type of contraction the force of the contraction is directly related to the size of the potential difference across the membrane of the smooth muscle cell. No further depolarization leading to an action potential occurs but the smooth muscle cell nevertheless contracts. Such tonic contractions without action potentials are found, for instance, in the proximal stomach.

◆ Long spike bursts during many slow waves. The smooth muscle cells generate action potentials during the depolarization phase (as usual) and during the hyperpolarization phase. The smooth muscle cells are contracted throughout this interval. Such long discharges of action potentials are observed in the colon amongst other regions.

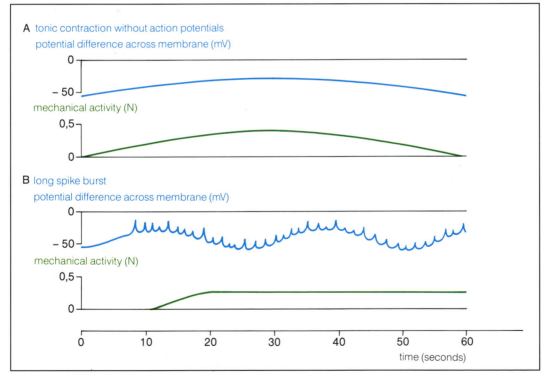

Figure 14: Tonic contractions in the gastrointestinal tract. A: Tonic contraction without action potential (spike-free); the force of the contraction is directly related to the size of the potential difference across the membrane. B: Long spike bursts: the action potentials occur throughout the cycle of potential fluctuations.

The alimentary canal in the fasting state

When the food (except the undigested particles) has passed through the small intestine, the movements of the stomach and intestines cease. This is called the **fasting, or interdigestive, pattern**. The stomach is quiescent for about 40 minutes, this interval being **phase I** of the interdigestive pattern. Thereafter peristaltic contractions are again gradually initiated, ushering in **phase II**, which also lasts about 40 minutes. Throughout this interval the frequency of the electrical control activity in the stomach is constant at 3 waves per minute. At the start of phase II there are few depolarizations that are coupled with a contraction. The number of such contractions increases rapidly; the frequency of the peristaltic contractions of the stomach rises steadily to a maximum of 3 waves per minute. The amplitude of the contractions also

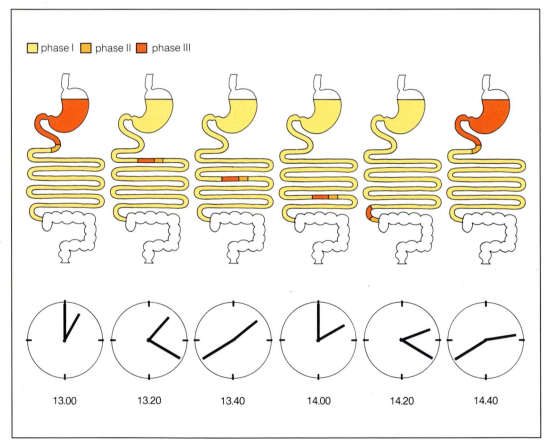

phase I phase II phase III

13.00   13.20   13.40   14.00   14.20   14.40

Figure 15: The MMC is gradually propagated through the gastrointestinal tract. About 1.5 hours after its start in the stomach it reaches the distal small intestine and the pattern begins again in the stomach.

continually increases. For about 10 minutes the contractions persist at the maximum frequency and force (**phase III**); in the stomach this rate is 3 waves per minute and the amplitude about 1.5 times that of the contractions of the full stomach. At this point the LOS pressure is at its highest (Figure 27, p. 70). Subsequently the contractions fade away. The stomach is again quiescent (phase I). This rhythmic pattern of gastric contractions is renewed about every 90 minutes. It is called the **interdigestive migrating motor complex** (MMC*). Generally the pylorus prevents the passage of particles of food greater than 0.5–1.0 mm in diameter. When the stomach is in phase III however, the contractions are so powerful and the pylorus opens to such an extent that larger undigestible food residues can pass. In the stomach and the proximal duodenum, phase III occurs at about the same time. In the fasting state, the maximum frequency in the duodenum is 12 contractions per minute. From the duodenum the MMC migrates distally at a speed of 5–10 cm per minute. After about 1.5 hours the MMC is able to reach the terminal ileum (Figure 15). Sometimes the contractions do not get so far and instead die out more proximally. Owing to the MMC, every 1.5 hours, the entire contents of the stomach and small intestine are swept away into the large intestine. The most important function of the MMC is to hold the small intestine free from stasis, thereby preventing bacterial overgrowth. Also during phase III in the stomach and proximal duodenum, gastric juice, bile and pancreatic juice are secreted (Figure 16). The MMC is thus a mechanical and chemical "broom".

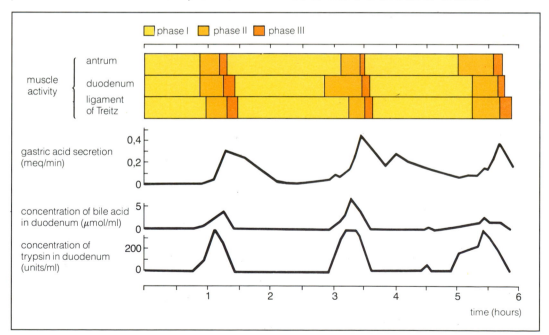

Figure 16: The MMC is a motor and secretion pattern.

* This is a motor and secretion pattern, but we shall follow convention and call it the migrating motor complex.

The alimentary canal after a meal

Immediately after the start of a meal the motility and secretion pattern of the digestive system alters: the postprandial pattern starts. The mere acts of seeing and chewing food constitute (via the brain) a stimulus that causes the stomach to contract. From the very beginning of a meal the proximal stomach undergoes tonic relaxations. In this fashion the stomach can accept food, and gastric pressure does not rise too much (Figure 38, p. 91). Right after the start of a meal, the distal stomach begins to contract phasically in irregular fashion. The contractions stabilize into a pattern within a few minutes:

3 contractions per minute (the frequency of the electrical control activity of the stomach) are conducted over the distal stomach. The contractions of the distal stomach are peristaltic from corpus to antrum. In this manner the food is gradually transported from the stomach to the duodenum and the small intestine. During and after a meal fairly irregular contractions are observed that are propagated over a short distance along the intestine. As a function of the consistency, composition and size of the meal, 1–5 hours can elapse before a fully digested meal leaves the stomach. Passage through the small intestine from duodenum to colon takes on average 1.5 hours. Subsequently the material can reside in the colon for 24–48 hours.

Patterns over the 24-hour cycle

Figure 17 gives an overview of the distribution of the postprandial and interdigestive periods of the stomach and intestines over the 24-hour cycle when three normal meals are eaten and a coffee and tea break are taken. Many people have more frequent consumption of, for example, soft drinks, biscuits and snacks. In this situation it is possible that the stomach and small intestine are in the postprandial state throughout the day.

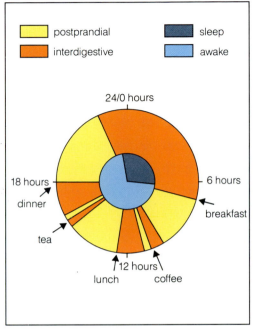

Figure 17: Whether the gastrointestinal tract is in the postprandial or interdigestive state depends on the intake of food. Shown here is an example of a 24-hour period in which three meals, one coffee and one tea break were taken.

From oesophagus to anus

The oesophagus

Problems related to swallowing and food passage can be caused by disturbances of the motility pattern of the oesophagus. Such disturbances can also induce "angina-like" pain.

Introduction

The oesophagus is not simply a tube through which food passes. It is an organ with its own movement patterns and its own innervation. Sometimes these movement patterns are disturbed. If that happens, swallowing becomes difficult or impossible, one chokes, or the food will not go down. Or angina-like retrosternal pain can develop. Oesophageal symptoms can be caused by gastro-oesophageal reflux (see Chapter 6). In general a thorough examination is necessary since the symptoms can point to serious disorders.

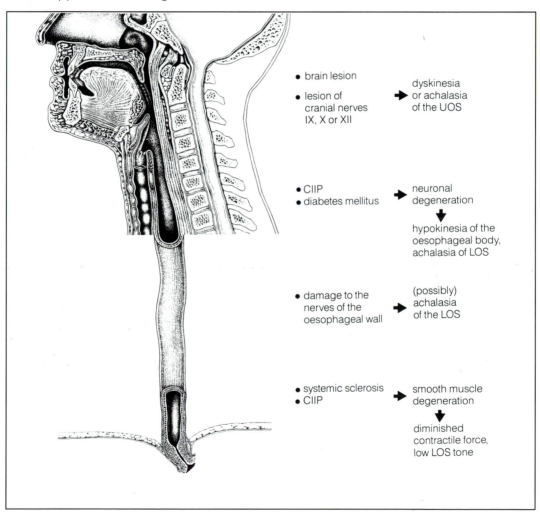

- brain lesion
- lesion of cranial nerves IX, X or XII
  → dyskinesia or achalasia of the UOS

- CIIP
- diabetes mellitus
  → neuronal degeneration
  ↓
  hypokinesia of the oesophageal body, achalasia of LOS

- damage to the nerves of the oesophageal wall
  → (possibly) achalasia of the LOS

- systemic sclerosis
- CIIP
  → smooth muscle degeneration
  ↓
  diminished contractile force, low LOS tone

Figure 18: Overview of the causes of disturbances of the movement pattern of the oesophagus.

The oesophagus and swallowing

The oesophagus at rest

At rest the oesophagus is tightly closed above and below. The upper oesophageal sphincter (UOS) consists of striated muscle tissue. This sphincter builds up a high pressure (40–120 mmHg [5–16 kPa]). The lower oesophageal sphincter (LOS) consists of smooth muscle tissue. This sphincter is also constricted at rest but it maintains a lower pressure (10–15 mmHg [1.3–2 kPa]). At rest the UOS and the LOS are constricted, so that gastric juices cannot get into the oesophagus or, more serious yet, the trachea or lungs.

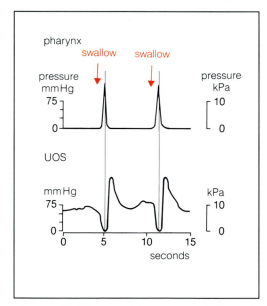

Figure 19: Manometric representation of normal swallow movements (schematic). A powerful peristaltic pharyngeal contraction coincides with a short relaxation of the UOS. This is followed by a more powerful contraction than at rest—the aftercontraction.

Swallowing

The entry of food into the hypopharynx elicits a swallow reflex. Swallowing is a co-ordinated pattern of relaxation and contraction of hypopharynx, UOS, oesophagus and LOS. In a normal

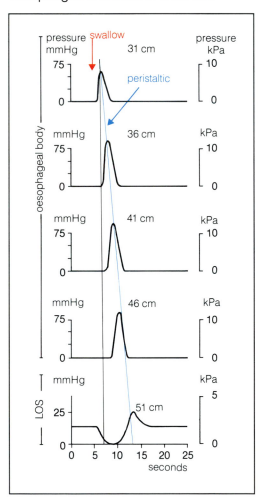

Figure 20: Manometric representation of primary peristalsis of the oesophagus (schematic). The swallow movement is followed by a contraction that is propagated distally and that coincides with a relaxation of the LOS, which lasts a few seconds.

swallow movement the hypopharynx contracts at the same time as the UOS relaxes (Figure 19). The UOS relaxes for 1–1.5 seconds. In the oesophageal body a peristaltic contraction occurs after the swallow movement and is propagated toward the stomach (Figure 20). Before the peristaltic contraction reaches the distal oesophagus, the LOS opens for a few seconds. The peristalsis observed with normal swallowing is called primary peristalsis. If gastric material flows back into the oesophagus (reflux), the oesophageal wall stretches and this also causes peristaltic movements—so-called secondary peristalsis. This type of peristalsis also coincides with a relaxation of the LOS. Secondary peristalsis can be experimentally induced by the blowing up of a balloon in the oesophagus.

Intermezzo 4
Examination of the oesophagus

◆ **Manometry** (p. 288) is the most important technique for identifying disturbed oesophageal motility. A standard manometric examination of the oesophagus takes about 20 minutes and causes the patient little inconvenience. Twenty-four-hour manometry is useful for recording disturbed movements even though they occur unpredictably and briefly only a few times per day. If appropriate one can attempt to provoke disturbed movements in the course of manometric recording.

◆ **Endoscopy** (p. 290) of the oesophagus is suitable for showing a stricture (consequent upon a tumour for instance) or an inflammation. Sometimes a spasm can be observed by means of endoscopy (Figure 23).

◆ **Radiography** (p. 283) is effective in detecting a stenosis or a foreign body. With cineradiography the contractions of the oesophagus during a swallow movement can be followed.

◆ **pH recording** (p. 293) is used when it is suspected that gastro-oesophageal reflux is a cause of the symptoms (Chapter 6).

Disturbances of the movements of the oesophagus

Each of the motor functions of the oesophagus is liable to disturbance and these disturbances can bring about severe symptoms. In history-taking it is important to differentiate between the following:

◆ **swallowing difficulties**, in which the patient has to make an effort to get the food to pass from the pharynx to the oesophagus (oropharyngeal dysphagia)

◆ **transit complaints**, in which the food passes with difficulty through the oesophagus (oesophageal dysphagia)

◆ **angina-like retrosternal pain attacks**, possibly consequent upon a motility disturbance of the oesophagus.

It is typical of a disturbance of the motility pattern of the oesophagus that both solid and liquid food pass poorly, whereas with an organic obstruction of the oesophagus, liquid food often passes easily.

Primary and secondary motility disturbances

A distinction is made between primary and secondary oesophageal dysmotility. With secondary motility disturbances another disease is involved (like systemic sclerosis or muscular atrophy) that is also attended by motility disturbances of the oesophagus. With primary motility disturbances the cause is unknown. The manometric pattern is sometimes characteristic, such as with oesophageal spasms, the nutcracker oesophagus or achalasia, but often anomalies are observed that are difficult to classify. Motility disturbances of the oesophagus are in fact rather rare. Unfortunately we cannot pronounce on their prevalence, which can be determined only after epidemiological manometric studies. To our knowledge, however, these have never been performed.

Primary disturbances of oesophageal motility

In examining a patient who presents with swallowing or passage complaints or with angina-like retrosternal pain, organic causes should first be excluded (Intermezzo 5, see also pp. 216 and 226) and then one examines the oesophageal motility.

Swallow disturbances

Once it has been established that the cause of a swallowing disturbance is not organic, one can examine whether it is due to a motility disturbance. Often the movements of the hypopharynx and the UOS are not attuned to one another. The most frequent anomaly is **dyskinesia of the UOS**, in which the sphincter does not open at the appropriate time. For example, it can close before the pharynx completes its contraction. Sometimes the UOS relaxes during swallowing in timely fashion but not wide enough. This disorder is called **achalasia of the UOS**. These anomalies cause swallowing difficulties and choking, sometimes together with aspiration pneumonia. The innervation of the UOS region is frequently defective in these patients. Disorders of the central nervous system, like cerebrovascular accidents or tumours, or impairment of cranial nerves IX, X or XII may be involved. Yet other neurological disorders may be observed. The swallowing disturbance can be so severe that the patient can be fed only by means of a tube. Sometimes myotomy of the UOS improves the situation.

**Intermezzo 5
Exclusion of other disorders**

Swallowing or passage difficulties and angina-like retrosternal pain can be provoked by motility disturbances of the oesophagus, but also by other serious disorders. Further examination is almost always necessary (Figure 107, p. 226).

◆ If a patient has difficulty swallowing or if food will not go down, a stricture or an inflammation in the hypopharynx or oesophagus can be responsible. Strictures can result from a tumour or from gastro-oesophageal reflux (peptic stricture). It is particularly important to exclude a **tumour**. To this end the patient can be referred to an ear, nose and throat specialist, an internist or a gastroenterologist; endoscopic or radiographic examination is necessary. Endoscopy is capable of revealing a peptic stricture, amongst other pathologies. Only after organic anomalies have been excluded can a functional examination of the oesophagus be considered.

◆ (Angina-like) retrosternal pain attacks can be caused by oesophageal dysmotility, but more often a **cardiac disorder** or **gastro-oesophageal reflux** is involved. Examination by a cardiologist is important to eliminate cardiological anomalies.

Achalasia (of the LOS)

When food cannot go down the oesophagus smoothly (oesophageal dysphagia) a manometric examination of the movements of this organ may be advisable. In a number of patients with oesophageal dysphagia a typical manometric profile is found: the LOS relaxes inadequately (achalasia of the LOS). In addition, in this disorder there are no peristaltic and only simultaneous contractions in the oesophagus (Figure 21). Both sexes are liable to this pathology at any age. The process begins insidiously. In the early stages it is difficult to make this diagnosis on endoscopic or radiological grounds. Sometimes it can be made only after many years. It is not uncommon for patients complaining of achalasia to be referred

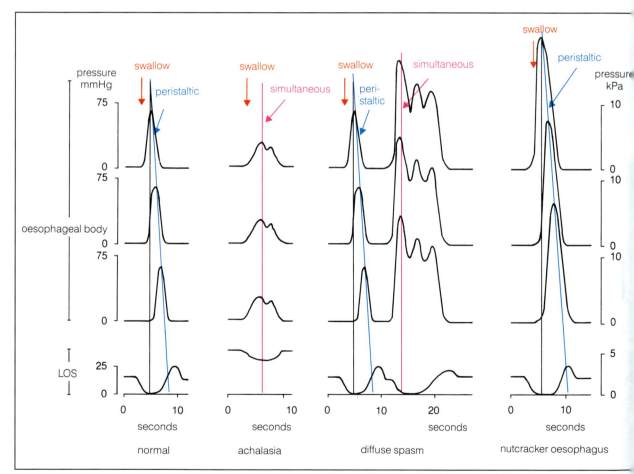

Figure 21: Schematic representation of the manometric profile in primary motility disturbances of the oesophagus: achalasia, diffuse spasms and nutcracker oesophagus.

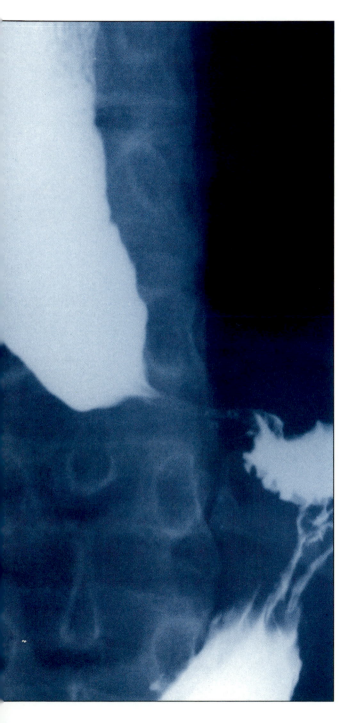

initially to a psychiatrist. In the advanced stages of the disease, radiological examination discloses a telltale picture (Figure 22). The oesophageal body is widened, normal peristaltic contractions are absent and the LOS is spastically constricted—the mouse tail appearance. The causes of achalasia are not yet known. Many researchers suspect impairment of the nerve fibres in the oesophageal wall or in the brain. Achalasia is preferentially treated by pneumatic dilation of the LOS. A balloon with a diameter of 30–40 mm is introduced endoscopically. Blowing this balloon up stretches the LOS. This procedure effectively reduces the LOS pressure. An alternative is surgery, i.e. Heller's myotomy.

Figure 22: Radiograph of the oesophagus in a patient with achalasia. The oesophagus is widened and contains a considerable quantity of old food residues. The lower oesophagus is spastically contracted. The so-called mouse tail appearance is evident.

Diffuse oesophageal spasms and the nutcracker oesophagus

If it is unlikely that a cardiological anomaly is responsible for angina-like retrosternal pain, pH-monitoring and manometry should be used to detect disordered reflux or motility. If the pain attacks are brought on by contractions of the oesophagus, this can, in principle, be demonstrated by manometry: during an attack excessively long-lasting and strong simultaneous contractions are observed, i.e. **diffuse oesophageal spasm** (Figure 21). The endoscopic profile of this disorder can be characteristic (Figure 23). Oesophageal spasm attacks are sometimes more or less predictably induced by emotion or food. On the other hand, some patients suffer from attacks rarely or unpredictably, so that diagnosis is difficult. If one suspects diffuse oesophageal spasm, one can attempt to provoke the abnormality by administering a cholinesterase inhibitor (e.g. edrophonium) or stretching the oesophagus with a balloon. Manometry can determine if the pain is accompanied by oesophageal spasm. In other patients with pain, oesophageal contractions can be observed that may be normally (peristaltically) propagated through the oesophagus but that display an abnormally high amplitude. This profile typifies the **nutcracker** oesophagus (Figure 21). The diagnosis of this disorder can be made only by means of manometry. The nutcracker oesophagus and diffuse spasm sometimes coexist. Angina-like pain can also result from **gastro-oesophageal reflux** (Chapter 6). 24-hour pH-monitoring is an effective way of excluding this disorder as the cause of the pain (p. 293). In the treatment of oesophageal spasm, it is important to explain the cause of the symptoms; once the patient becomes aware that the pain arises from the oesophagus and not the heart, he or she is reassured and finds it easier to tolerate the attacks. Further, drugs can be used that relax the smooth muscle tissue. Examples are nitroglycerin or calcium antagonists like diltiazem or nifedipine. In some patients pneumatic dilation can also be performed. Exceptionally, a long myotomy of the oesophagus can be done.

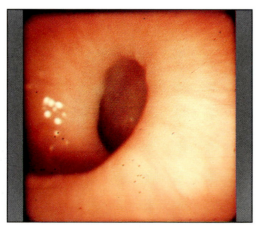

Figure 23: Endoscopic image of an oesophagus with diffuse spasms. Such coil-like spasms are seldom observed endoscopically. (Reproduced with permission, from Dr H. Poen, Utrecht.)

Aspecific motility disturbances

In a fairly large proportion of patients with disordered transit or angina-like retrosternal pain, manometry reveals a disturbed oesophageal motility pattern. When this pattern is not typical of achalasia, oesophageal spasms or the nutcracker oesophagus, the term aspecific motility disturbances is used. A disordered oesophageal motility pattern is also observed with symptom-free persons, but only occasionally. Elderly persons frequently present symptoms due to dysmotility, the term for this disorder being presby-oesophagus. The treatment of aspecific dysmotility is often a matter of trial and error. Explanation and reassurance are important. If the oesophageal contractions are too strong or they last too long, one can attempt to relax the smooth muscle with nitroglycerin or calcium antagonists like diltiazem or nifedipine. If, on the other hand, the contractions are too weak, one should adopt a strategy of stimulating oesophageal motility with prokinetic drugs like cisapride, domperidone or metoclopramide (cf. Chapter 14). That these drugs have a clear effect in patients with aspecific motility disturbances has not been established in double-blind trials. Nevertheless a number of patients are satisfied with the results of these treatments.

Secondary disturbances of oesophageal motility

Oesophageal dysmotility frequently occurs secondarily to a number of diseases. In general this type of dysmotility is caused by **systemic sclerosis** (Figure 24). When this disorder

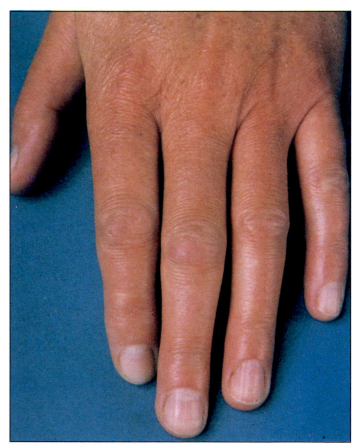

Figure 24: The characteristic appearance of the skin in systematic sclerosis. (Photograph reproduced with permission, from J. v.d. Stek, Rotterdam.)

affects the oesophagus, peristalsis in the lower two-thirds of the organ is gradually weakened (Figure 25). In the upper two-thirds, in which striated muscle is the major component of the wall, peristalsis often persists intact. The

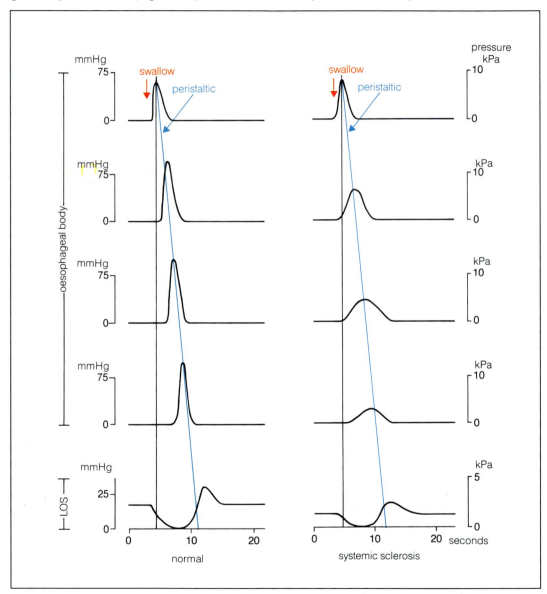

Figure 25: The manometric profile in scleroderma in comparison with the normal situation (schematic). Propagation is normal but the amplitude of the contractions in the distal oesophagus is diminished. LOS pressure in systemic sclerosis is generally low.

LOS pressure is decreased in this disorder, which can bring about reflux symptoms. One aspect of **diabetes mellitus** is degeneration of the intramural neurons (neuropathy). A progressive neuropathy also occurs in the gastrointestinal system (p. 246). In many patients with long-running diabetes, oesophageal dysmotility sets in secondarily, which, however, generally gives rise to few symptoms. Secondary disordered oesophageal motility is also frequently found in rare diseases, such as **muscular dystrophy** (p. 250) or **chronic idiopathic intestinal pseudo-obstruction** (CIIP, p. 243). In CIIP dysmotility can be found in all portions of the digestive tract, the cause of which is unknown. With this secondary dysmotility the movements of the oesophagus are either too weak or not frequent enough. It is then attempted to stimulate oesophageal motility and tone by means of prokinetic drugs. It has been established that cisapride promotes the movements of the oesophagus in patients with systemic sclerosis, muscular dystrophy and diabetes.

Conclusion

In a number of disorders of the digestive tract the general practitioner is able to make a diagnosis and begin treatment on the basis of history-taking and a physical examination. This is not advisable when dealing with oesophageal dysmotility since its symptoms can point to other, more serious, disorders—like tumours or cardiological anomalies—which must be excluded first by means of supplementary examinations. With oesophageal dysmotility, making an accurate diagnosis is a matter of no mere academic importance. The disorders may be rare, but their diagnosis has a crucial impact on treatment.

Chapter 6

Gastro-oesophageal reflux disease

Heartburn, belching and acid regurgitation are complaints frequently met in general practice. They point in the direction of gastro-oesophageal reflux. Reflux can bring about oesophagitis, sometimes with serious complications. How do you determine whether your patient has abnormally vigorous reflux and how serious are the consequences of such reflux? How do you treat a patient with reflux symptoms?

Introduction

It has recently come to light that gastro-oesophageal reflux can occur without our being aware of it. Sometimes it is accompanied by discomfort: a burning sensation behind the sternum or a sour taste in the mouth. The pain can become severe; inflammation of the oesophageal mucosa (oesophagitis) or other serious complications can develop. Whether gastric material flows back into the oesophagus depends on the tone of the lower oesophageal sphincter (LOS) and the intra-abdominal pressure. Normally the LOS is constricted and in this way it prevents reflux from the stomach. With each swallow the LOS opens briefly, thus facilitating passage of the food bolus. However, even without a swallow the LOS sometimes opens in both healthy and diseased persons. When this happens, gastro-oesophageal reflux occurs (physiological reflux). A disordered LOS motility can bring about pathological reflux.

In addition, the refluxed gastric material can be eliminated from the oesophagus too slowly, which can also lead to symptoms. Delayed gastric emptying can also play a role in gastro-oesophageal reflux.

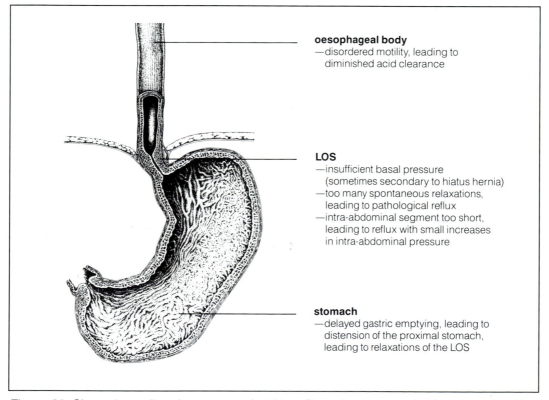

oesophageal body
—disordered motility, leading to diminished acid clearance

LOS
—insufficient basal pressure (sometimes secondary to hiatus hernia)
—too many spontaneous relaxations, leading to pathological reflux
—intra-abdominal segment too short, leading to reflux with small increases in intra-abdominal pressure

stomach
—delayed gastric emptying, leading to distension of the proximal stomach, leading to relaxations of the LOS

Figure 26: Sites where disturbances can lead to reflux symptoms and reflux oesophagitis.

Normal movements of the LOS

The LOS is usually constricted

The function of the LOS is to keep the acidic gastric juice in the stomach. The LOS is usually constricted but the LOS pressure fluctuates considerably.

◆ After a meal the LOS pressure is lower than it is on average in the fasting state. The postprandial LOS pressure is determined by the type of food that one has eaten: food, alcohol and nicotine lower the LOS pressure transiently (Table 2); protein-rich food significantly raises the LOS pressure.

◆ When the stomach is empty, the interdigestive migrating motor complex (MMC, p. 46) is active. This periodic pattern can also be observed in the LOS activity (Figure 27).

◆ The LOS pressure is affected by endogenous hormones. Progesterone, for example, lowers the LOS pressure. This explains why, in the second half of the menstrual cycle and during pregnancy, there is more reflux.

◆ Finally, the LOS pressure can be influenced by drugs (Table 3).

Because the LOS pressure changes "spontaneously", the phrase "'the' basal LOS pressure" is inappropriate. It follows that a single measurement of the LOS pressure can provide misleading information. In order to obtain relevant information on the activity of the LOS one must record it over long periods as well as in the fasting state and after a meal.

Spontaneous relaxation of the LOS

In recent years it has been discovered that there are also (apparently spontaneous) longer-lasting relaxations of the LOS. These spontaneous relaxations do not coincide with swallowing and they last on average about 20 seconds (Figure 28). In healthy persons these spontaneous relaxations occur on average 20–30 times per day. They are more likely to arise when the stomach is full. In this way gases can escape from the stomach. Thanks to the development of the Dent sleeve (p. 289) it has become possible to measure the LOS pressure during a longer interval. Only with the arrival of this device was it possible to discover the spontaneous relaxations of the LOS. Although these are termed "inappropriate", this adjective has more to do with the lack of understanding by the research worker

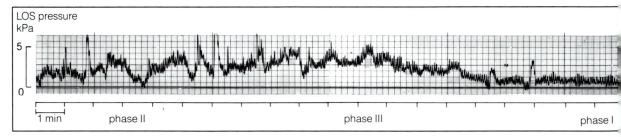

Figure 27: The LOS pressure during the interdigestive migrating motor complex (in the fasting state). During phase III of this complex the LOS pressure peaks.

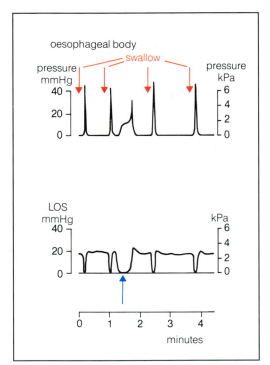

Figure 28: Manometric representation of a spontaneous LOS relaxation (arrow). The other relaxations coincide with the peristaltic contractions of the oesophageal body.

than the relaxations themselves. During these relaxations the barrier to reflux from the stomach to the oesophagus is absent, thus enabling acidic gastric contents to flow into the oesophagus (gastro-oesophageal reflux), which then becomes acidic (Figure 29). Under normal conditions the oesophagus responds by propagating peristaltic waves, which transport the gastric juices back into the stomach. In healthy persons it has been established that almost all reflux episodes result from a spontaneous relaxation. Only occasionally does reflux occur in healthy volunteers

fat	peppermint
chocolate	caffeine
alcohol	nicotine

Table 2: Food, food ingredients and stimulants that lower the LOS pressure.

- anticholinergic agents (or drugs with anticholinergic side-effects)
- β-adrenoceptor agonists (isoprenaline)
- theophylline
- benzodiazepines
- calcium blockers (verapamil, nifedipine, diltiazem)
- opiates

Table 3: Classes of drugs that lower the LOS pressure.

under normal LOS pressure. Generally (with an intact oesophagus) a reflux episode is not noticed as long as the gastric contents do not reach the oral cavity.

Normal (physiological) and pathological reflux

Notwithstanding, too many spontaneous relaxations of the LOS can occur or the gastric juices can reside too long in the oesophagus. If more than 50 reflux episodes per 24 hours occur or if the pH of the oesophagus is lower than 4.0 for more than 1 hour, reflux is regarded as pathological. If the oesophageal wall is damaged the acidic gastric juices can stimulate pain sensors, with the inevitable result that the reflux is perceived. This happens more often with pathological reflux. However:

- pathological reflux does not always manifest itself by symptoms;
- physiological reflux can also produce symptoms;

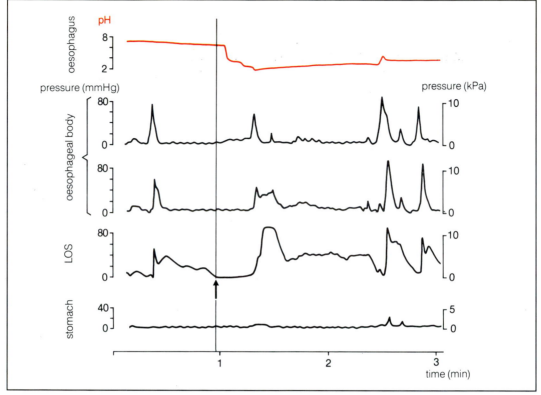

Figure 29: Gastro-oesophageal reflux during "spontaneous" LOS relaxation. Such a relaxation starts at the arrow. Shortly thereafter the pH in the distal oesophagus drops (red). Then secondary peristaltic waves travel down the oesophagus to clear it. (Reproduced with permission, from Dent 1987.)

◆ chronic pathological reflux does not always cause oesophagitis;

◆ in some persons oesophagitis develops without pathological reflux and without reflux symptoms;

◆ occasionally oesophagitis is accidentally discovered in a patient who has not presented any reflux symptoms but in whom an endoscopy was performed (for other reasons).

Diagnosis: pathological reflux

History

In taking the history of a (suspected) reflux patient it is important to focus on the type of symptoms he or she presents and on when these occur.

◆ What are the symptoms?
The symptoms consist of a burning sensation (pyrosis) behind the sternum or high in the epigastrium, generally called heartburn by the patient. Sometimes small quantities of gastric contents reach the mouth (regurgitation). In addition gastro-oesophageal reflux can bring on retrosternal pain attacks. These attacks can bear a striking resemblance to angina pectoris or a heart infarct.

◆ When do the symptoms occur?
Both the times at which the symptoms appear and the circumstances surrounding them can be important sign-posts.
— Are the symptoms mainly observed during the day or at night?
— Are they experienced predominantly while the patient is lying, bending or straining?
— Do they tend to occur after a meal?
— Are they related to a particular type of food?
— Is the patient on drugs (Table 3)?
— Does the patient suffer from coughing or dyspnoea attacks at night?

Diagnostic guidelines are given on p. 228.

Intermezzo 6
Hiatus hernia?

With hiatus hernia of the oesophagus the opening in the diaphragm through which the oesophagus passes is too wide. Part of the stomach then protrudes into the chest cavity. The terms "hiatus hernia", "reflux disease" and "reflux symptoms" are sometimes used to denote the same disorder. That is unfortunate, for after all, only one in three patients with a hiatus hernia has oesophagitis and, on the other hand, only about half of patients with oesophagitis have hiatus hernia. It is believed that disturbances of the LOS function sometimes develop secondarily to hiatus hernia. How this happens is not yet clear. In any case, whether or not it is established that a patient has hiatus hernia has **no implications** for treatment. The hiatus hernia itself does not give rise to symptoms. In general it is not advisable to upset patients with a hiatus hernia with a remark that they have a hernia of the diaphragm.

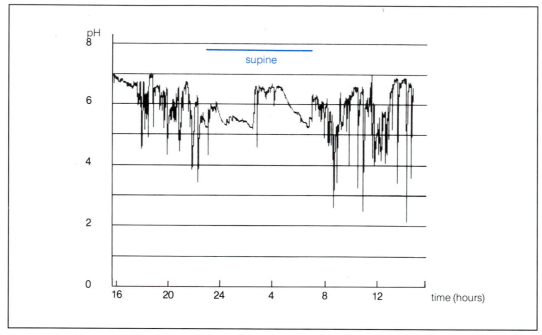

Figure 30: 24-hour pH curve of healthy volunteer: upright reflux episodes (during the day), no reflux episodes while supine at night.

24-hour pH recording

As a technique for demonstrating and quantifying gastro-oesophageal reflux, 24-hour pH recording in ambulatory patients is more suitable than any other.* The pH measured in the oesophagus is usually neutral (5.5–7.0). Sometimes however the pH falls sharply (Figure 30). Such a drop indicates that reflux has occurred. The total time during which the pH remains below 4.0 is an important parameter. In the pH analysis a distinction is made between night reflux, when the patient is in the lying position, and day reflux, when the patient moves about, sits or stands. Pathological day reflux is shown in Figure 31A. With night reflux the oesophagus generally remains acidic for a long period (Figure 31B). The patient can press a button during monitoring to indicate that he or she is experiencing a symptom. In this way it can be established if the patient's symptom is really related to reflux (Figure 31A). Especially when symptoms are atypical or when there is no reflux oesophagitis, 24-hour pH recording can furnish crucial information.

*By means of pH recording reflux of acidic gastric juices can be measured. But if the refluent is not acidic it cannot be reliably established by pH recording whether reflux has in fact occurred. This can be the case if the acid secretion has been inhibited with high-dose H_2-blockers or omeprazole or if the contents of the small intestine (with a neutral or alkaline pH) have flowed back to the oesophagus. The contents of the small intestine can also damage the oesophageal wall. It is generally assumed however that that such reflux plays a role in the development of oesophagitis only after removal of the distal stomach (Billroth resection) or the whole stomach.

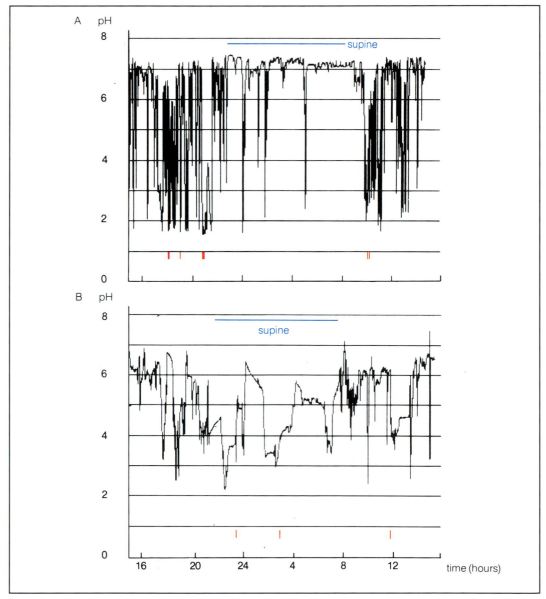

Figure 31: 24-hour pH curve. A: Pathological upright reflux. The red lines indicate the times at which the patient had reflux symptoms. These events all coincide with a drop of the pH to below 4. The symptoms of this patient are clearly caused by reflux.
B: Pathological reflux during sleep. During sleep in particular the oesophageal pH persists too long at a low value; brought about by disordered oesophageal clearance.

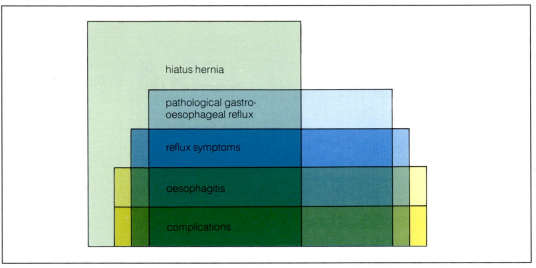

Figure 32: Schematic overview showing how the concepts applied to gastro-oesophageal reflux disease relate to and overlap with one another.

Intermezzo 7
Definitions and concepts

◆ Reflux symptoms include heartburn, regurgitation and belching; angina-like retrosternal pain attacks also occur in this context.

◆ The term **physiological reflux** is used if the reflux episodes are usually short and infrequent during sleep There may not be more than 50 such episodes over 24 hours, and the pH of the oesophagus may not be less than 4.0 for longer than 1 hour over 24 hours.

◆ The term **pathological reflux** is used if there are more than 50 reflux episodes over 24 hours, and/or the pH is less than 4.0 for more than 1 hour over 24 hours. On the one hand these conditions do not necessarily produce symptoms and on the other, even if reflux is normal there can be reflux symptoms.

◆ **Oesophagitis** is an inflammation of the mucosal membrane of the distal oesophagus such as seen by means of endoscopy and a biopsy.

◆ **Gastro-oesophageal reflux disease** (GORD) is often adopted as an umbrella term to catch reflux symptoms that may or may not be further examined or specified.

◆ The term **hiatus hernia** (diaphragmatic hernia) is used to refer to an abnormal protrusion of part of the stomach into the chest cavity. Hiatus hernia can be identified by radiographic or endoscopic examination.

◆ By **complications** of oesophagitis are meant bleeding, stenosis of the distal oesophagus owing to the formation of fibrous tissue, and Barrett's epithelium.

Figure 32 presents an overview.

**Intermezzo 8
Investigation of gastro-oesophageal reflux**

In the determination of gastro-oesophageal reflux, 24-hour pH recording is the most logical and reliable method. The times of reflux episodes are variable and unpredictable.

◆ Only **24-hour pH recording** gives a full picture of gastro-oesophageal reflux; the other diagnostic techniques have the drawback of discrete registration. We shall now briefly mention these techniques.

◆ **Radiographic examination** is not reliable enough to disclose abnormal gastro-oesophageal reflux. It is capable however of evidencing severe oesophagitis (but not the mild form of the disorder). A radiograph can also detect a hiatus hernia.

◆ **Endoscopy** cannot be used to observe reflux itself, although it is an ideal technique for ascertaining the sequelae of oesophagitis. (The different grades of oesophagitis are defined by means of endoscopy.) This method can also reveal hiatus hernia.

◆ With the aid of **isotope techniques** reflux of a radio-labelled test meal can be measured. This method is also less suitable than 24-hour pH recording. In fact, it is hardly used any more.

◆ In the **standard acid reflux test** a standard quantity of acid is introduced into the stomach. Then short-term pH recording is used to determine if (abnormal) reflux occurs. Also with this technique, the short duration of measurement is the chief disadvantage.

◆ In the **Bernstein test** the pH of the distal oesophagus is artificially lowered by perfusion of an acidic solution. The doctor checks whether the patient can identify his or her own symptoms. The same information can be obtained in a more physiological manner by means of 24-hour pH recording.

The consequences of reflux

The acidic gastric contents can damage the wall of the oesophagus. In the first stage small local inflammations develop, but these can enlarge. Chronic reflux can give rise to complications: ulcer, stricture or metaplasia of the mucosal membrane. How can the damage to the oesophageal wall be ascertained?

Examination of the sequelae of reflux

Endoscopy is the recommended method for studying the effects of gastro-oesophageal reflux on the mucosal membrane of the oesophagus. A flexible endoscope is used, with the aid of which both mild and severe effects of reflux can be viewed. Endoscopy is the "gold standard" for diagnosing oesophagitis. A radiographic examination is suitable for identifying the advanced stages of oesophagitis but not the early stages. Furthermore, with endoscopy the damaged tissue can be biopsied. After biopsy, reflux oesophagitis can be firmly differentiated from tumour or other forms of oesophageal inflammation.

The stages of oesophagitis

The severity of endoscopically observable reflux oesophagitis is conventionally divided into grades. The most frequently used classification is that of Savary and Miller (Figure 34).

◆ grade I: the erosions are isolated and do not extend over the full circumference of the oesophagus (Figure 34A)
◆ grade II: the erosions are confluent but do not extend over the full circumference of the oesophagus (Figure 34B)
◆ grade III: the erosions cover the full circumference of the oesophagus (Figure 34C)
◆ grade IV: there are complications, like ulcer, peptic stricture or Barrett's metaplasia (Figures 34D, E, F).

Complications of oesophagitis

In chronic oesophagitis connective tissue can form in the wall of the oesophagus, narrowing its lumen. Such a "peptic" stricture can cause dysphagia. Peptic strictures are generally short and are found regularly directly above the juncture between the oesophageal and gastric mucosal membrane (Figure 34E). As a result of chronic reflux oesophagitis, metaplasia of the oesophageal epithelium can develop. If it does, an epithelium forms that resembles gastric or small intestinal

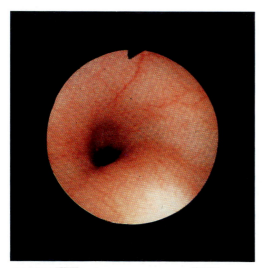

Figure 33: Endoscopic image of a normal oesophagus. (Reproduced with permission, from Prof. G.N.J. Tytgat, AMC.)

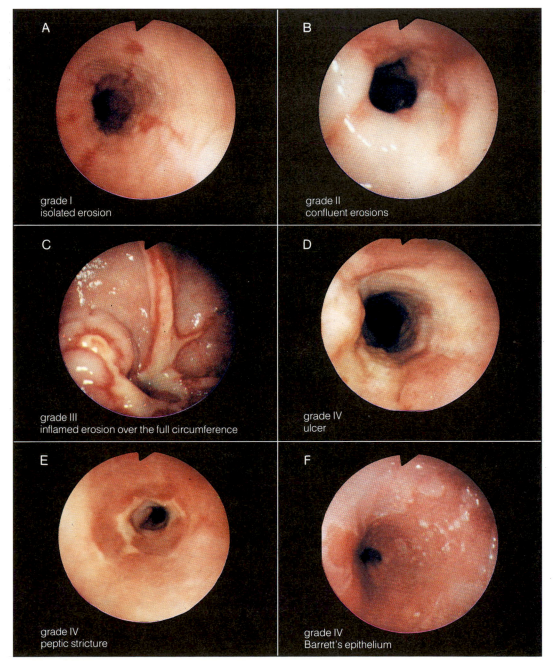

Figure 34: Endoscopic images of the stages of oesophagitis. (Reproduced with permission from Prof. G.N.T. Tytgat, AMC.)

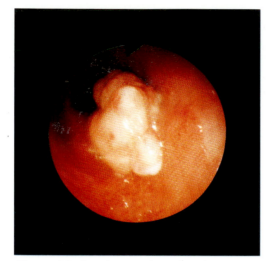

Figure 35: Carcinoma that developed in Barrett's epithelium. (Reproduced with permission, from Prof. G.N.T. Tytgat, AMC.)

The origin of pathological reflux

Reflux symptoms are generally provoked by gastric juices (acid and pepsin). And yet, as a rule, an overproduction of gastric acid is not involved. Rather, the gastric juices end up at the wrong site of the LOS. Due to what dysfunction is it that too much gastric juice ends up in the oesophagus or stays there too long? Pathological reflux can be detected by pH recording. The origin of such reflux remains unclear, however, if one limits oneself to this technique. If the cause is to be investigated, the pressure in the oesophagus, LOS and stomach must be measured, i.e. one needs manometry.

epithelium. This epithelium is called Barrett's epithelium, after its discoverer. Macroscopically Barrett's epithelium can be identified by the proximal location of the mucosal juncture (Figure 34F). It is important to identify Barrett's epithelium since carcinomas (adenocarcinoma) can develop in it (Figure 35). Annual endoscopic examination of patients with Barrett's oesophagus is therefore recommended.

Disturbances of the oesophageal body

When acid gets into the oesophagus, under normal circumstances it is rapidly expelled by secondary peristalsis to the stomach (Figure 29). However, in some patients with reflux oesophagitis the amplitude of the oesophageal contractions is too small. In other patients simultaneous rather than peristaltic contractions occur. These anomalies result in inadequate acid clearance and overexposure of the oesophagus to the acid. It is entirely conceivable that this dysfunction of motility can cause damage to the oesophageal wall. The reverse mechanism is also possible: oesophagitis disturbs the oesophageal peristalsis.

Disturbance of the LOS

The LOS constitutes the most important barrier against reflux. An obvious possibility therefore is that abnormal gastro-oesophageal reflux develops as a result of dysfunctional activity of the LOS. Since 1976 it has been possible to perform long-term, reliable measurement of the LOS pressure (with the Dent sleeve, p. 289). Accordingly we now know much more about normal and disturbed LOS functioning.

◆ In about 40% of patients with reflux disease "the" basal LOS pressure is too low, so that when the intra-abdominal pressure rises, reflux can easily occur. In other patients however the basal LOS pressure is normal or even relatively high.

◆ In many patients with pathological reflux the number of spontaneous relaxations of the LOS is high. In this situation reflux develops without an increase in the intra-abdominal pressure (compare Figure 29).

In some patients we see a combination of a low basal LOS pressure and a high rate of spontaneous relaxations of the LOS. The normal position of the stomach is under the diaphragm. On average 60% of the LOS lies within the abdomen. When the intra-abdominal pressure rises, the LOS closes extra tightly. This is a safety mechanism against reflux consequent upon an increase in the intra-abdominal pressure. It functions properly only if the stomach is normally positioned and less well if there is a hiatus hernia. There is also evidence that a hiatus hernia can bring about dysfunctioning of the LOS.

Disturbances of the stomach

In some patients with reflux oesophagitis, gastric emptying is slow; it is possible that a sluggish stomach plays a role in the genesis of gastro-oesophageal reflux; it is evident that if gastric emptying is slow the stomach will distend. The basal LOS pressure, in turn, will fall and the number of spontaneous LOS relaxations will increase. After removal of the distal stomach or the whole stomach the contents of the small intestine can flow to the oesophagus. This can seriously damage the oesophageal wall.

The treatment of pathological reflux

In the treatment of gastro-oesophageal reflux disease modifications of lifestyle, drugs and surgical procedures can be used (Table 4).

Modification of lifestyle

A number of patients with reflux symptoms can benefit from some simple modifications of their lifestyle.

◆ For supine reflux it can be useful to elevate the head of the bed by placing blocks about 10 centimetres high under the bedposts.

◆ Upright reflux can sometimes be decreased only if the patient wears loose clothes and avoids straining, lifting and bending; it should be remembered that all these factors raise the intra-abdominal pressure.

◆ Overweight persons sometimes experience an improvement after weight reduction. Some patients with reflux symptoms appear to have a critical body weight; if they are too heavy they suffer symptoms.

◆ If stimulants and certain foods are avoided, reflux symptoms can be curbed; nicotine, coffee, chocolate, alcohol, citrus fruits, peppermint and fatty foods increase the likelihood of reflux.

◆ Certain drugs lower the LOS pressure (Table 3). Anticholinergic agents have this effect, but so do drugs with anticholinergic side-effects. The latter group can often be replaced by drugs with a single desired action without the anticholinergic side-effects. Also,

---

Lifestyle modifications
— elevate head of bed (blocks under bedpost, no extra pillow)
— lose weight
— quit smoking
— avoid tight clothing
— avoid straining and bending
— avoid eating before going to sleep
— avoid coffee, alcohol and chocolate
— stop LOS-lowering drugs

Drug therapy
— acid reduction
— promotility
— mucosal protection

Endoscopic dilation of strictures

Surgery
— Nissen procedure
— Belsey procedure

Table 4: Treatment of reflux disease.

non-anticholinergic drugs can induce reflux symptoms. In this case, one should then ask oneself whether a particular drug cannot be replaced or avoided.

Drug therapy of reflux symptoms

In the treatment of reflux symptoms (or reflux oesophagitis) three strategies are available: attack the gastric acid, protect the mucosa or stimulate motility. **Gastric acid secretion** is reduced by H_2-blockers or an H^+/K^+-ATPase-blocker (omeprazole, p. 259). Omeprazole inhibits gastric acid secretion much more potently than H_2-blockers. There are currently four different H_2-blockers: cimetidine, ranitidine, famotidine and nizatidine. For acute relief of symptoms antacids can be used. In oesophagitis sucralfate **protects the oesophageal mucosa**. This substance adheres to protein-rich surfaces like the substrate of an ulcer. A coating forms on the ulcer or the erosion, as a result of which the mucosa is given the chance to repair itself. Three **prokinetics** are available: cisapride, domperidone and metoclopramide (p. 260). All three motility drugs reduce symptoms but cisapride has the most potent action. It has been established only for cisapride that it promotes healing of oesophagitis. In the treatment of reflux oesophagitis one takes into account the severity of the disorder and the type of therapy, i.e. acute or maintenance.

◆ Patients with relatively mild heartburn can be treated with prokinetics, antacids or both. If the symptoms are not eliminated, H_2-blockers can be administered for a few weeks.

◆ For the acute treatment of grade III or IV oesophagitis the choice is between omeprazole and a combination of cisapride and a high-dose H_2-blocker. Sometimes sucralfate is added to this combination.

◆ If the object is to prevent relapse, often a maintenance treatment of oesophagitis is desirable. The effect of a maintenance treatment with a conventional dose of an H_2-blocker is disappointing. However, high-dose therapy with these drugs does lower the relapse rate. There is evidence that cisapride also prevents relapse. The use of a prokinetic is inherently more logical than long-term treatment with H_2-blockers. In severe relapse it is sometimes necessary to opt for a maintenance treatment with omeprazole.

Dilation of peptic strictures

Peptic **strictures** in the oesophagus can generally easily be dilated. A metal **guide wire** is passed through the stricture using an endoscope. A silicone prosthesis, the diameter of which increases evenly to about 16 mm, is then passed over the guide wire. Such dilations can often be performed on an out-patient basis without anaesthesia. Finally, when the stricture is dilated, its cause, namely pathological reflux, must also be treated.

Surgery in oesophagitis

In what situations is surgery desirable in oesophagitis?

1. Some patients object strongly to the idea of long-term medication; they prefer an operation.
2. With H$_2$-blockers or omeprazole the pain and symptoms due to gastric acid often disappear but a number of patients still suffer from regurgitation of the (now non-acidic) gastric contents*. Sometimes the regurgitation is so annoying that an operation is desirable.
3. Some oesophagitis patients do not respond adequately to drugs.

Various **surgical techniques** to combat gastro-oesophageal reflux have been described (Table 4). Placement of an Angelchick prosthesis to prevent reflux has become obsolete because of numerous complications. Nowadays Nissen's operation (Figure 122, p. 274) is generally performed. In this technique the upper part of the stomach is folded like a cuff around the LOS. This operation can decrease reflux spectacularly, the reflux of gastric contents to the oesophagus often being completely inhibited.

With anti-reflux operations, however, complications are rather frequent and some of them are irreversible. Accordingly strict **indications and contra-indications** are now observed with this type of surgery. Crucial in this respect is the pathophysiological basis of the symptoms and the oesophagitis (cf. Figure 26, p. 69).

1. If diminished acid clearance is a major cause of the symptoms, one should be reluctant to perform this operation.
2. If over-frequent gastro-oesophageal reflux is a major cause of the symptoms and the oesophagitis, the operation has the greatest chance of success. The pathological reflux can be determined only by 24-hour pH monitoring which reveals the strength of the relationship between the occurrence of symptoms and drops in pH. One is inclined to operate only after 24-hour pH monitoring shows that pathological reflux is accompanied by a reasonably normal acid clearance. This reluctance should be all the stronger when there are symptoms but no oesophagitis.
3. If delayed gastric emptying is a major cause of the symptoms and the oesophagitis, one tends not to proceed with the operation.

Previously the diagnosis of patients with reflux symptoms was often based exclusively on X-rays. Thanks to a more accurate formulation of indications and improved surgical technique, anti-reflux surgery is now often successful, even in the longer term.

* Cisapride decreases regurgitation (as expected) more than H$_2$-blockers or omeprazole.

Conclusion

The sequelae of abnormal gastro-oesophageal reflux can vary from mild symptoms to serious complications due to reflux oesophagitis. On the basis of the clinical history, the general physician must determine for each patient whether supplementary examinations are appropriate and, if so, which ones. In many patients who consult a general physician about reflux symptoms these are relatively mild: most can benefit from simple life-style and dietary adjustments. If these measures are not adequate, short-term use of cisapride, antacids, sucralfate or H_2-blockers is often effective. There is, however, a group of patients with severe symptoms who do not respond very well to treatment. For them a combination of cisapride and high-dose H_2-blockers can be used, or gastric acid secretion can be more potently inhibited with omeprazole and, if desired, cisapride. It is important to identify a stricture since dilation of it on an out-patient basis is effective against dysphagia. It is important to diagnose Barrett's epithelium since this predisposes for the development of adenocarcinoma.

References

Dent J. A new technique for continuous sphincter pressure measurement. Gastroenterology 1976; 71:263–267

Dent J. Recent views on the pathogenesis of gastro-oesophageal reflux disease. Baillière's Clin Gastroenterol 1987; 1: 727–745

Dent J. e.a. Mechanisms of lower oesophageal sphincter incompetence in patients with symptomatic gastrooesophageal reflux. Gut 1988; 29:1020–1028

Dodds WJ, e.a. Pathogenesis of reflux oesophagitis. Gastroenterology 1981; 81:376–394

Fisher RS, e.a. The lower esophageal sphincter as a barrier to gastrooesophageal reflux. Gastroenterology 1977; 72:19–22

Galmiche JP, e.a. Combined therapy with cisapride and cimetidine in severe reflux oesophagitis: a double blind controlled trial. Gut 1988; 29:675–681

Klinkenberg-Knol EC, Jansen JMBJ, Festen HPM, Meuwissen SGM, Lamers CBMW. Double-blind multicentre comparison of omeprazole and ranitidine in the treatment of reflux oesophagitis. Lancet 1987; 1:349–351

Richter JE, Castell DO. Gastrooesophageal reflux-pathogenesis, diagnosis and therapy. Ann Intern Med 1982; 97:93–130

Tytgat GNJ, Nicolai JJ, Reman FC. Efficacy of different doses of cimetidine in the treatment of reflux oesophagitis. Gastroenterology 1990; 99:629–634

FROM OESOPHAGUS TO ANUS

Stomach, pylorus and proximal duodenum

The motility of stomach, pylorus and proximal duodenum can now be measured objectively in patients. Symptoms that were previously considered to be primarily psychogenic are now known to be attended by a verifiable disordered motility of the stomach and duodenum. Examination of gastric emptying and of gastric and duodenal motility can be necessary for correct diagnosis and an optimal approach.

88

Introduction

Thanks to new investigational techniques much has been discovered recently about the activity of the stomach, pylorus and duodenum. The movements of these parts are more complex than had been thought previously. Moreover, these movements must occur in concert if the food is to be transported properly.

If the movements of stomach, pylorus and duodenum are disordered, upper abdominal symptoms can result, like nausea, upper abdominal pain, early satiety and anorexia. In patients with lower abdominal symptoms, gastric and duodenal motility can now be objectively recorded. It is also now possible to measure concrete dysmotility in connection with symptoms that were formerly considered to be psychogenic. Examination of gastric emptying and the motility of stomach and duodenum can be necessary for correct diagnosis and the elaboration of an optimal strategy. Upper abdominal symptoms are often caused by abnormal movements of the stomach.

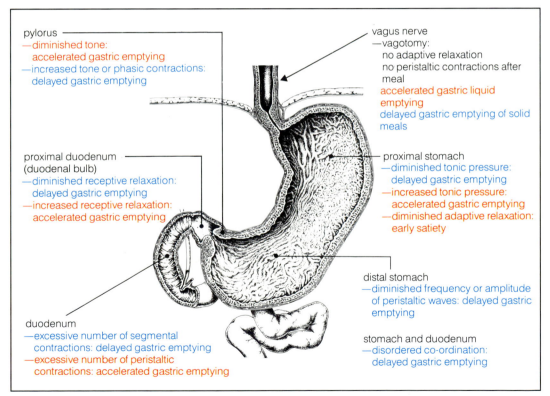

Figure 36: Schematic representation of disturbances of movements of the stomach, pylorus and duodenum.

Gastric motility

The movements of stomach, pylorus and proximal duodenum

During and after the meal the stomach and intestines present a motility and secretory pattern (the postprandial pattern) that is different from the one observed some hours after the meal (the pattern of the fasting state, cf. p.46). Because storage, digestion, transport and absorption are the most important functions of the stomach and intestines, we shall first discuss the postprandial pattern and then the fasting pattern. The motility patterns of the upper and lower parts of the stomach are different. The following regions are differentiated from one another:

◆ the proximal stomach: the fundus and the proximal part of the corpus
◆ the distal stomach: the distal part of the body and the antrum.

The proximal stomach after a meal

The best known gastric movements are the mixing peristaltic contractions. These are found in the distal but not in the proximal stomach. The proximal stomach shows only tonic activity. The intra-abdominal pressure is carefully regulated.

◆ **Receptive relaxation.** Immediately after a swallow the proximal stomach relaxes for about 20 seconds (Figure 37). Thus when food passes into the stomach, the pressure drops briefly. In this way the stomach "receives" a particle of food.
◆ **Adaptive relaxation.** When food arrives in the stomach, the intra-abdominal pressure tends to rise. It must not rise too much however, for

if it did, the gastric contents would enter the small intestine too quickly, or, if the LOS were incompetent, they would flow back to the oesophagus (Chapter 6).

By means of a control system the intra-abdominal pressure is kept at the appropriate level. In response to a small increase in the intra-abdominal pressure, stretch sensors in the stomach are activated, and via a vago-vagal reflex these ensure that the smooth muscle of the proximal stomach relaxes. This activity is called adaptive relaxation (Figure 38). In this manner intra-abdominal pressure is well regulated. The adaptive relaxation of the proximal stomach facilitates the reservoir and the propulsive functions of the stomach. If

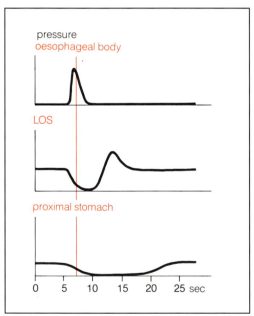

Figure 37: The proximal stomach relaxes in order to receive the food: receptive relaxation. This phase lasts about 20 seconds.

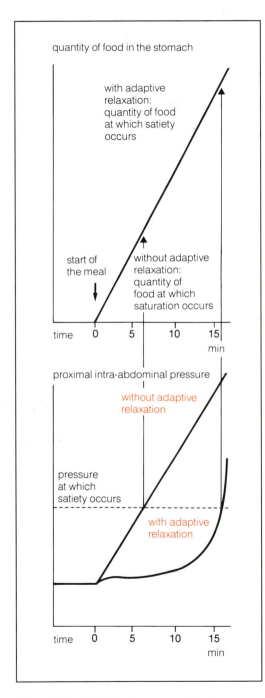

quantity of food in the stomach

with adaptive relaxation: quantity of food at which satiety occurs

start of the meal

without adaptive relaxation: quantity of food at which saturation occurs

time   0   5   10   15|
                         min

proximal intra-abdominal pressure

without adaptive relaxation

pressure at which satiety occurs

with adaptive relaxation

time   0   5   10   15
                        min

the pressure rises above a critical value, a feeling of fullness is experienced. Without adaptive relaxation the intra-abdominal pressure would shoot up during a meal and a sensation of satiety would be experienced too early (Figure 38). This early satiety occurs after certain vagotomies (truncal or highly selective, Figure 123, p. 275).

The distal stomach during and after the meal

Whether during, after or between meals, the muscle cells of the stomach display their electrical control activity of three depolarizations per minute. Sometimes these depolarizations are attended by contractions, depending on the meal or the phase of the MMC (p. 46). Immediately after the start of a meal, the stomach begins to produce peristaltic contractions. Initially it contracts only during some depolarizations, in irregular fashion. Within a few minutes of the start of the meal a stable pattern of contractions occurs: three contractions per minute travel through the stomach. The contractions of the distal part of the stomach correspond to phasic, peristaltic waves that traverse only this part of the stomach. The contractions of the stomach are always peristaltic, from corpus to antrum.* These peristaltic movements arise as a result of, amongst other things, stimuli from stretch sensors in the stomach and the stimulation is

Figure 38: When food enters, the proximal stomach relaxes in order to maintain a sufficiently low pressure. This activity is called adaptive relaxation and it lasts several minutes.

---

* It is not likely that simultaneous contractions occur. As far as we know, objective measurements have not yet disclosed "gastric spasms". Even in vomiting there are no antiperistaltic contractions of the stomach. Very rarely an ectopic pacemaker is found in the antrum of patients which has a frequency of more than three contractions per minute. However, this ectopic pacemaker can induce contractions that travel from antrum to corpus. They can bring about severe nausea and vomiting.

conducted via the vago-vagal reflex path. The function of these movements is the mixing and grinding of solid food. As a result of the peristaltic movements the food is transported to the pylorus.

The pylorus after a meal

It was previously thought that the pylorus remained tight shut most of the time and opened only sporadically. The reality is just the opposite: most of the time the pylorus is partially open and only sporadically is it closed. The muscle of the pylorus contracts in such a way that a small canal remains open. Through this, liquids and small food particles pass on condition that there is a pressure gradient between stomach and duodenum. This gradient results in either gastric emptying or duodenogastric reflux. When the

organism is in the fed state, the pylorus is affected by the antrum and duodenum.

◆ **Influence of the stomach**. As a peristaltic wave from the antrum approaches the pylorus, the latter closes, propelling the food back forcefully toward the mouth (Figure 39). Only a small quantity of liquid chyme can leave the stomach before the pylorus closes. Depending on the composition of the meal, about 1–4 ml of chyme per contraction reaches the duodenum in humans.

◆ **Influence of the duodenum**. When the concentration of carbohydrate, protein or fat in the duodenum is too high, sensors are intensely stimulated, causing the pylorus to close (see below). The pylorus then produces a pattern of rhythmic

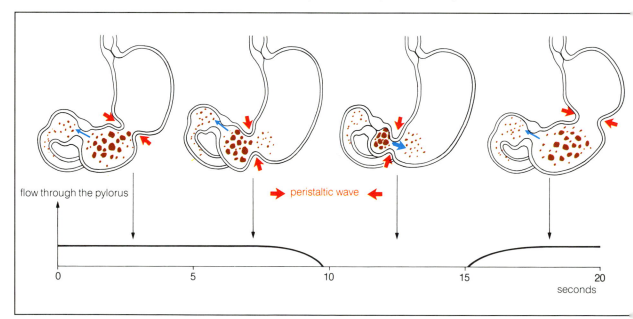

Figure 39: Flow of the gastric contents during a peristaltic contraction of the distal stomach.

contractions, mostly at the frequency of the antral contractions (3 per minute), sometimes at that of the duodenal contractions (12 per minute) and sometimes at that of a combination of the frequency of contraction of the two. It follows that the small intestine cannot be overloaded with calorie-rich food.

Intermezzo 9
Normal duodenogastric reflux?

Previously it was believed that the pylorus remained shut most of the time and that reflux from the duodenum to the stomach was involved in the genesis of gastritis and gastric ulcer. We now know however that the pylorus is mostly open. This can be shown clearly by means of manometric and ultrasonographic monitoring. It has also been established that there are episodes of duodenogastric reflux in asymptomatic healthy persons. Reflux occurs in both the fasting and the fed state. Despite these advances, no effective methods have been devised for recording reflux to the stomach over a long interval. The current assumption is that only after a stomach operation is reflux from duodenum or small intestine to the stomach so extensive that the mucosa of the stomach or duodenum is damaged.

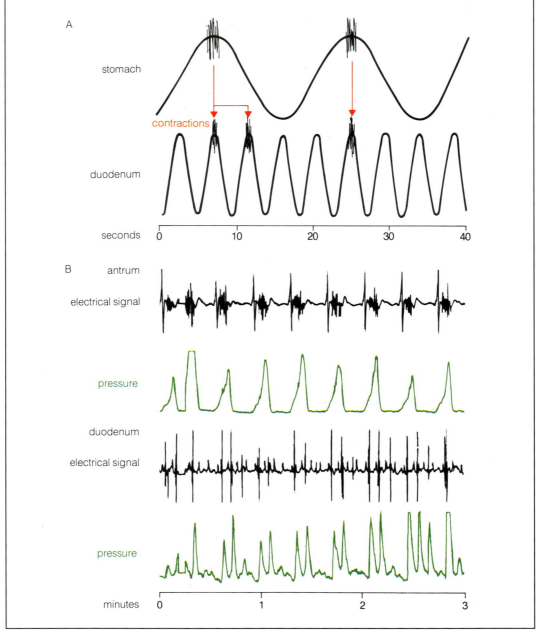

Figure 40: Co-ordination of antrum and duodenum. A: The principle of antroduodenal co-ordination: a contraction in the antrum increases the probability of a contraction in the duodenum. B: Measurement of antroduodenal co-ordination.

Stomach and duodenum after a meal

In humans three peristaltic waves per minute travel through the distal stomach after the meal. This is the maximum frequency for the stomach. In principle the duodenum can contract 12 times per minute, but after a meal there are fewer contractions. The contractions of stomach and duodenum are generally co-ordinated; only when a peristaltic wave reaches the pylorus does the smooth muscle in the duodenum contract. This is what is meant by antroduodenal co-ordination (Figure 40). Duodenal contractions occur only upon depolarization of the smooth muscle. Depolarizations in the duodenum are four times as frequent as those in the antrum. Sometimes the duodenum contracts once and sometimes several times after a contraction in the antrum. Antroduodenal co-ordination probably plays an important part in normal gastric emptying.

Movements in the fasted state

Above, the movements of stomach, pylorus and proximal duodenum were described as a reaction to food. However some time after the meal they show another pattern: the MMC. When all the food except the undigestible particles have passed out of the small intestine, the movements of stomach and duodenum cease. For about 40 minutes the stomach is quiescent (phase I). Then peristaltic contractions gradually resume (phase II). This phase also lasts about 40 minutes. All this time the electrical control activity in the stomach continues at three depolarizations per minute. At the beginning of phase II, few depolarizations coincide with a contraction. The number of these coincidences increases rapidly; the frequency of gastric peristaltic contractions rises steadily to a maximum of three waves per minute. The amplitude of the contractions also increases steadily. For about 10 minutes the contractions continue to occur at the maximum frequency and force (phase III). In the stomach this frequency is three waves per minute and the amplitude is about 1·5 times that of the contractile waves of the postprandial stomach. After this phase the contractions fall off again and the stomach is again quiescent (phase I). The MMC is repeated about every 90 minutes. Generally the pylorus prevents the passage of food particles greater than 0.5–1.5 mm in diameter. Only in phase III can larger indigestible food residues pass through the pylorus. In the duodenum the phases of the MMC occur later than in the stomach. In the fasted state too the maximum frequency in the duodenum is 12 contractions per minute.

Gastric emptying

All these movement patterns of the stomach, pylorus and duodenum serve to transport the food, in appropriate quantities, in the right direction. Thanks to radioisotopic studies, we now know much better how long it takes for the constituents of food to pass from the stomach to the intestines.

Gastric liquid emptying

After a liquid meal, the food leaves the stomach at an approximately exponential rate (Figure 41). The transit time depends, amongst other factors, on the osmotic and calorific value of the meal (see below). For healthy volunteers the mean half-time is 20 minutes for a 10% glucose solution. Emptying of a liquid meal begins immediately. Generally, some 300 ml of liquid can be evacuated from the stomach in a mean time of 30 minutes.

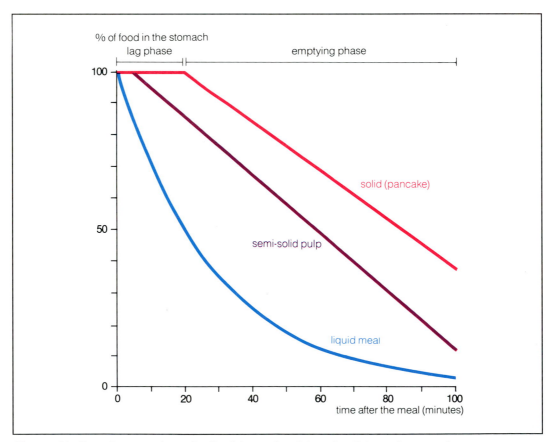

Figure 41: Gastric emptying of a liquid, semi-solid and solid meal: normal curves.

Gastric emptying of a solid meal

After a solid or a semi-solid meal the food begins to leave the stomach only after some minutes (Figure 41). This delay is called the lag phase. When the food actually passes out of the stomach, the post-lag phase begins. Per unit of time then, a mean fixed quantity of food is evacuated from the stomach; gastric emptying is more or less linear with time. The lag phase for a semi-solid meal is shorter than that for a solid meal. The effect of consistency was studied in the following investigation. Healthy volunteers ate a semi-solid meal consisting of a given quantity of pulp and a solid meal consisting of a pancake containing an equal quantity of calories, carbohydrate, protein and fat. For the pulp the lag phase was 5 minutes and for the pancake 22 minutes (Figure 41). The explanation of these results is that the stomach first had to convert the pancake into a semi-solid. On average the stomach requires 1 hour to eliminate a light meal consisting of bread and something to drink and 3 hours for a somewhat more elaborate hot meal.

Intermezzo 10
Investigation of gastric emptying

The gastric emptying rate of liquid and solid food (and its transport time through the intestine) can be determined by different techniques.

◆ **Radioisotopic techniques**. The "gold standard" for investigating gastric emptying is scintigraphy (p. 286). In this connection various test meals are used, ranging from liquid to solid. Liquid meals are labelled with the isotope [111]Indium-DTPA and solid meals with a [99m]Technetium-tin colloid. The gastric emptying and the intestinal filling time can be measured with a gamma camera (Figure 127, p. 286).

◆ **Radiographic examination**. Radiography is less suitable for the determination of gastric emptying. It is not clear, for example, whether barium sulphate stays homogeneously mixed in the food. It is suspected that this substance sometimes leaves the stomach more rapidly than the food and sometimes more slowly. However, radiography is perfectly capable of revealing severe gastric retention.

◆ **Intubation**. A dye is injected into the stomach and a sample of the gastric and duodenal contents is taken at different time points with a catheter that has been inserted into these parts. In this way it is possible to measure the gastric emptying and gastric acid secretion simultaneously. The method is complex, however, and is therefore used exclusively in research.

◆ **Ultrasonography**. With ultrasound the gastric liquid emptying can be measured more or less quantitatively. However, this technique requires much experience and has accordingly been limited to research activities until now (see also Figure 132, p. 292).

Control of gastric and pyloric motility

The role of the extrinsic and intrinsic nervous system

◆ Extrinsic innervation from the central nervous system ensures receptive and adaptive relaxation and activates the postprandial patterns of gastric motility. The effects of the central nervous system are clear after vagotomy: these patterns become disturbed and the frequency and amplitude of the contractions are diminished.

◆ Owing to the enteric nervous system (ENS), the stomach and intestines can perform many motor functions themselves. The MMC is characterized by a contractile and secretory rhythm that is generated by the intrinsic nervous system. This system also co-ordinates the movements of the individual parts of the digestive tract. In addition, it determines the tone of the stomach and intestines and make segmental and peristaltic contractions possible.

The influences of the extrinsic and the intrinsic nervous system are not always easy to identify. For example, a given function sometimes fails immediately after a vagotomy. It could be concluded from this event that this function is controlled by the vagus, but after some time this function can reappear without innervation of the vagus.

Hormones also have a clear effect on the gastrointestinal tract. Motilin, which, in the fasting state, plays a major role in gastrointestinal motility, is secreted by the duodenum.

The effect of food on gastric emptying

Food is complex, being characterized by a number of variables: quantity, consistency, the presence of particles, osmolarity, calorific content, and composition (carbohydrates, proteins, fats, vitamins, etc.). All these factors affect gastric emptying.

◆ The **volume** of the food. It was mentioned earlier that stretch sensors in the stomach elicit adaptive relaxation in the proximal stomach and peristaltic contractions in the distal stomach.

◆ The **osmolarity** of the food. Liquids with the same osmolarity as that of the body fluid (i.e. isotonic liquids) are transported most rapidly into the duodenum. Gastric emptying is slower with hypertonic and hypotonic liquids. (Figure 42). This activity is regulated by osmosensors in the duodenum. It is possible that gastric emptying is slower for hypertonic and hypotonic liquids in order to prevent unnecessary osmotic stress in the intestine. (The role of osmolarity was investigated in a study with liquids whose calorific content was zero so that the effect of this variable could be eliminated—see below.)

◆ The **composition** of the meal. Only a limited quantity of carbohydrate, fat and protein can be absorbed per unit time by the small intestine. If the stomach delivered these substances more rapidly, they would reach the small intestine only partially absorbed and as a result they would be converted by yeasts or bacteria (fermentation). Moreover unnecessary food would be lost. In order to adapt the gastric emptying to the absorption capacity of the small intestine, there are chemosensors in the duodenum that detect amino acids (amongst others, L-tryptophane), sugars, fats and pH. Mediated by neurons and hormones (amongst others, cholecystokinin) they diminish gastric contractility and induce the pylorus to contract. In this way they delay gastric emptying (Figure 43). In addition, they provoke the replacement of peristaltic contractions in the proximal duodenum by segmental contractions. They thus lengthen the time available for food absorption in the duodenum.

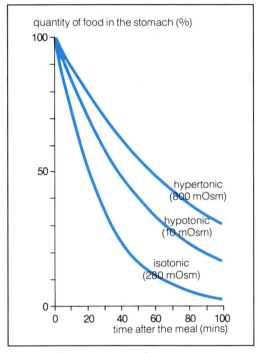

Figure 42: The effect of osmolarity of the food (zero calorific content) on gastric emptying: isotonic liquids empty most rapidly, hypertonic and hypotonic foods more slowly.

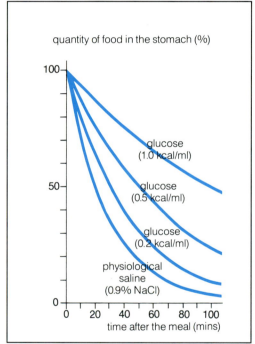

Figure 43: The effect of the calorific content of a liquid on gastric emptying. Gastric emptying is shown for liquids of different calorific content.

◆ The **size of the particles** in the food. Only small food particles can pass through the pylorus after a meal. Often a portion of the food must be broken down in the stomach into finer particles. The effect of particle size can be easily observed if the gastric emptying of pieces of liver is compared with that of liver that is ground into fine particles (homogenized) (Figure 44). Homogenized liver leaves the stomach almost like a liquid, whereas pieces of liver (1 cm across) create a lag phase. The other extreme is seen with indigestible pellets (7 mm in diameter): in the fed state all of these stay in the stomach, and in phase III of the MMC they are eliminated en masse (Figure 44).

◆ **The pH of the duodenum**. Per peristaltic wave of the stomach 0.5–2 ml of chyme passes through the pylorus. This substance is collected in the much larger duodenal bulb and there neutralized by the pancreatic juice. If the pH of the duodenum is transiently too low, gastric emptying is inhibited by the pH sensors in the duodenum. In this way the pancreas is given time in which to neutralize the acid chyme.

The result of all these activities is that the stomach conveys a fairly constant flow of energy to the duodenum (on average 8.5 kJ [2 kcal per minute]). How this entire process is regulated by sensors, nerves, hormones and muscle remains to be investigated in detail.

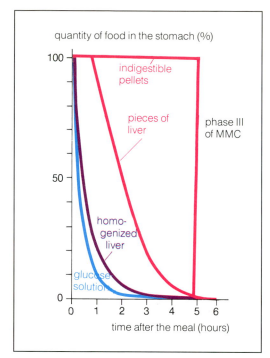

Figure 44: The effect of particle size on gastric emptying. Digestible pieces of food must first be broken down into tiny particles before they can be evacuated. Indigestible particles leave the stomach only during phase III of the MMC.

Intermezzo II
Investigation of gastric movements

There are different methods of studying gastric movements.

◆ **Intraluminal manometry**. The variations in the intragastric and intraduodenal pressure can be measured with perfused catheters or with pressure sensors. In this way the pressure can be measured at several points at the same time. To determine the intrapyloric pressure the Dent sleeve must be used (p. 289).

◆ **Electrogastrography** (EGG). The electrical activity (ECA and ERA, Chapter 4) of the stomach can be measured by placing electrodes on the upper abdomen (Figure 134, p. 294). An analysis of these findings provides an overview of the electrical control activity (Figure 53, p. 110). The EGG shows that after a meal, frequency slightly decreases and thereafter slightly increases. In this way irregularities concerning the electrical control activity are revealed (dysrhythmias, tachygastrias).

◆ **Ultrasonography**. After the patient has drunk a standard quantity of liquid (often 300 ml), the movements of stomach, pylorus and duodenum can be clearly observed (Figure 132, p. 292). If one studies the ultrasonograms on a screen for about 15 minutes, one is able to form an impression of the pattern of contractions of the antrum, pylorus and proximal duodenum. Moreover, it is possible to establish a relationship between the contractions of the antrum, pylorus and duodenum and the flow through the pylorus in both directions.

Motility disturbances of stomach, pylorus and proximal duodenum

Nausea, a feeling of fullness or bloatedness, pain in the upper abdomen, heartburn and similar symptoms often result from gastric dysmotility. What causes this dysmotility? In a number of patients it can be established that primary or secondary diseases disorder the functioning of the muscles and nerves of the stomach and intestines. In many other patients however, no cause can be found. We then speak of "idiopathic" disturbances.

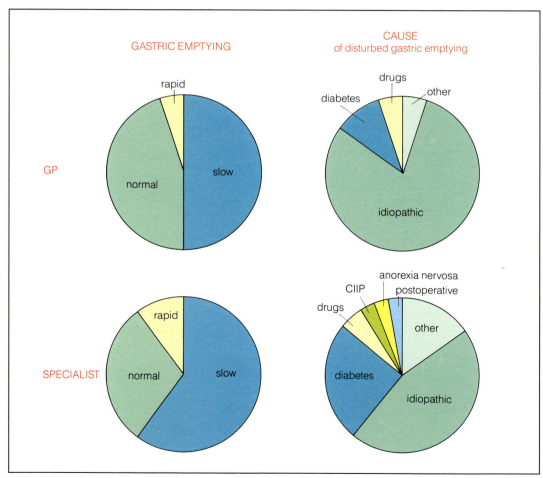

Figure 45: These disturbances are prevalent in patients with abdominal symptoms (without ulcer) for which the general physician is consulted. This figure is intended to give an impression only and not absolute proportions, the data for these not being available.

How does a doctor examine a patient with upper abdominal complaints? First organic disease, like peptic ulcers, gastric carcinoma, gall stones, pancreatitis, etc., must be ruled out. Then it may be necessary to investigate the gastric emptying and motility of the stomach and duodenum. It is sometimes too hastily concluded that upper abdominal symptoms are generally psychogenic. Examination, however, often shows that disordered gastric emptying is the cause. Thanks to gastric function tests, a doctor can now gain insight into the cause of gastric dysmotility, and with these methods can also evaluate the effects of drug therapy and surgery quantitatively.

Symptoms of gastric dysmotility
A disturbance of the contractions of stomach and duodenum may result in delayed or accelerated gastric emptying. Delayed emptying is much more common than accelerated (Figure 45). Guidelines for the diagnosis of

patients with dyspeptic symptoms and/or upper abdominal complaints are given on p. 218 and the following pages. The diagnostic problem consists in the fact that the symptoms of rapid and delayed gastric emptying are largely the same (Figure 46). These symptoms are: nausea, vomiting, belching, bloated/full feeling, early satiety, upper abdominal pain, heartburn, anorexia and sometimes weight loss. When gastric emptying is too rapid, in addition to these symptoms the dumping syndrome occurs. Vasomotor symptoms (pale skin, perspiration, fast pulse, or fainting) are seen 15–30 minutes after the meal. Occurrence of the dumping syndrome is a strong indication that the patient suffers from accelerated gastric emptying. It is important to differentiate between delayed and accelerated gastric emptying because treatment is different.

Disorders
Many disorders also manifest themselves in digestive tract dysmotility. In addition, pregnancy, immobilization or use of certain drugs can lead to gastrointestinal motility disturbances. Figure 36 gives an overview of the disturbances of parts of the stomach, pylorus and proximal duodenum and of the effects these disturbances can have on gastric emptying. Figure 45 gives an overview of the most frequently occurring disorders in connection with disturbed gastric emptying. A more elaborate overview is provided in Tables 9 and 10 (pp. 220 and 221).

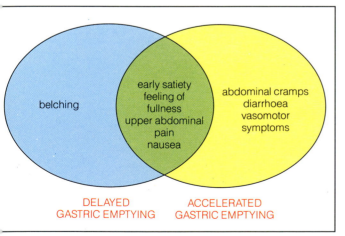

Figure 46: The symptoms of slow and accelerated gastric emptying.

Idiopathic gastroparesis

In a large group of patients with dyspeptic symptoms no organic cause can be found, so that the term "non-ulcer" dyspepsia is applied. Examination reveals that about half of these patients have delayed gastric emptying, especially of solid food (Figure 47). If gastric emptying is slow, further examination (manometry or electrogastrography, EGG) often discloses hypomotility of the antrum. In this case, the term idiopathic gastroparesis is used. In patients with idiopathic gastroparesis the electrical control activity is often disordered. During intervals of abnormal electrical control activity of the stomach, the contractions are infrequent (hypomotility) or absent (atony) in the antrum. In a number of patients

*Helicobacter pylori** can be isolated from the stomach (cf. p. 219).

Diabetic gastroparesis

In patients with diabetes mellitus, nerve fibres are often affected (neuropathy, p. 246). If this happens to nerve fibres in the stomach, gastric motility is disturbed and diabetic gastroparesis results. In these patients the tonic contractions of the proximal stomach are too weak in the fed state and the peristaltic contractions of the antrum are not frequent enough or are too weak (hypomotility of the antrum). Often the tonic and phasic contractions of the pylorus are slightly too strong. As a consequence of this complex of factors, gastric solid and liquid emptying are slow (Figure 48). In diabetic patients abnormal contractile patterns are also found in the fed state.

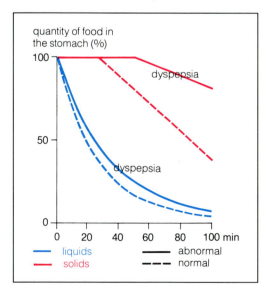

Figure 47: Gastric emptying curves for solid and liquid meals in dyspeptic patients.

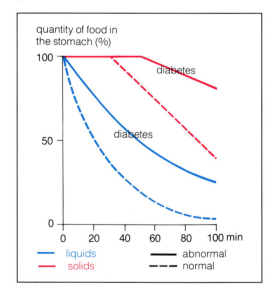

Figure 48: In patients with diabetic gastroparesis gastric emptying of solid and liquid meals is very slow.

* Until recently this bacterium was called *Campylobacter pylori*.

In particular, phase III of the MMC does not occur in the stomach. This is just the phase in which large, difficult-to-digest or indigestible food particles can leave the stomach. In some patients with diabetic gastroparesis these large particles leave the stomach very slowly; if appropriate, the patient can be advised to grind his or her food finely or chew it longer than usual. Unlike in the stomach, in the small intestine of diabetes patients, phase III of the MMC is intact. In a number of patients with diabetes mellitus a disordered gastric emptying can explain the poorly regulated blood sugar levels. Since gastric emptying is disturbed, food absorption is of course also impeded. Elaborate diets are not very effective as long as food absorption is disturbed. Treatment of the dysmotility enhances regulation of the blood sugar.

Intermezzo 12
Anorexia nervosa

Anorexia nervosa is generally considered to be a psychiatric condition. In addition to a resistance to eating, weight loss and amenorrhoea, patients with this disorder often complain of a feeling of fullness or bloatedness and early satiety at meals. Previously it was assumed that these gastrointestinal symptoms were psychogenic. Rather unexpectedly, however, researchers found that in some patients with anorexia nervosa, gastric emptying was disturbed (Figure 49). Manometry and EGG showed that there were gastric rhythm disturbances in these patients. Which disorder is primary in them, the psychic disturbance or the dysmotility? It is conceivable that dysmotility develops as a result of the chronic undernourishment in anorexia nervosa. But the resistance to eating could also be caused by the dysmotility, in particular by the unpleasant sensation after the meal.

In some patients with anorexia nervosa, cisapride accelerates gastric emptying, thereby controlling some of the symptoms. It seems likely that in some patients with anorexia nervosa, gastric dysmotility contributes to the clinical picture.

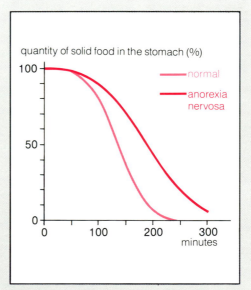

Figure 49: In some patients with anorexia nervosa gastric emptying of a solid meal is slow.

Gastric ulcer and duodenal ulcer

In patients with a gastric ulcer gastric solid emptying is generally slow, whilst liquids are evacuated at the normal rate (Figure 50). Manometric examination reveals that in patients with a gastric ulcer the antral contractions are generally too infrequent or too weak (antral hypomotility). Is the dysmotility caused by the ulcer or the ulcer by the dysmotility? Once the ulcer heals, in a fraction of the patients motility remains disturbed. Apparently in some patients the gastric ulcer is primary and in others the dysmotility is primary. In patients with duodenal ulcer, semisolids and liquids

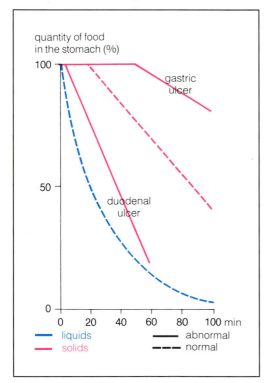

Figure 50: Gastric emptying curves for solid meals in patients with gastric and duodenal ulcer.

are eliminated much more rapidly than normal; the lag phase is shorter or even absent (Figure 50). It appears that their stomach does not differentiate between semisolids and liquids.

Motility disturbances after stomach operations

After a stomach operation new problems involving the stomach can arise. Globally, the following complications can ensue: slow or accelerated gastric emptying and pathological reflux of the contents of duodenum and small intestine into the stomach.

◆ After a Billroth-II gastric resection (Figure 124, p. 277) a portion of patients experience vasomotor symptoms, a feeling of fullness, and nausea and vomiting after the meal. Another group of patients is symptom-free. In B-II patients with symptoms semisolids are evacuated much more rapidly than in patients without symptoms (Figure 51). In B-II patients without symptoms the gastric emptying rate is the same as that in patients with duodenal ulcer.

◆ After vagotomy (whether intentional or unintentional) symptoms often develop (Figure 123, p. 275). The action of the vagus nerve induces adaptive relaxation of the proximal stomach after a meal and stimulates peristaltic contractions of the distal stomach. The disturbances after vagotomy are attributable to this fact. After vagotomy, gastric liquid emptying is too fast. When a vagotomized patient drinks, no adaptive relaxation occurs, the intra-abdominal pressure rises and

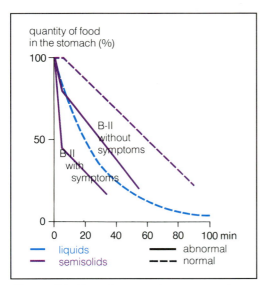

Figure 51: Gastric emptying curves for semisolid meals in patients who have had a B-II resection, with or without symptoms after the operation.

liquids are propelled out of the stomach too rapidly. After a solid meal, the stomach produces either no or too few peristaltic contractions; solid food is ground, mixed and transported too slowly, so that gastric emptying is too slow. A frequently used method of avoiding delayed gastric emptying after vagotomy consists of combining vagotomy with pyloroplasty (p. 275), as a result of which the resistance of the pylorus is diminished. After a truncal vagotomy with pyloroplasty semisolid meals are evacuated from the stomach too rapidly in the first 10 minutes, whilst solid meals are sometimes evacuated too rapidly but generally too slowly (Figure 52). If evacuation of solid meals is too

slow, a dilemma arises: solids leave the stomach too slowly and (semi)liquids too rapidly, so is it advisable to stimulate gastric motility or not? In some patients experimenting with semisolids of variable consistency yields favourable results: with food of a given consistency, symptoms stay within limits. In other patients another operation is indicated, in particular the Roux-en-Y operation, in which a small residual stomach is left (Figure 124, p. 277).

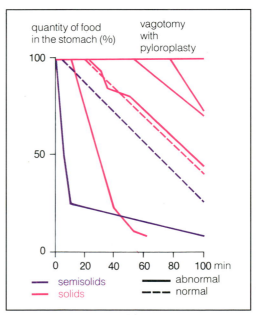

Figure 52: Gastric emptying curves for semisolid and solid meals in patients who have had a truncal vagotomy with pyloroplasty and experienced symptoms after the operation. Curves are given for five patients for emptying of solid meals because the differences between patients are substantial.

Bile reflux after stomach operations

Formerly it was thought that reflux of alkaline duodenal contents to the stomach could damage the mucosa. The pylorus was believed to constitute a barrier to this reflux. Now it is known that the pylorus is open most of the time and thanks to a new technique (the HIDA scan, p. 287) it is known that some reflux of bile into the stomach is normal. It is now assumed that only after a stomach operation is duodenogastric reflux severe enough to damage the gastric mucosa, so that only in this situation does pathological duodenogastric reflux arise. In healthy volunteers (who have not had gastric surgery) there is usually some, non-noxious duodenogastric reflux (i.e. physiological reflux). Nevertheless it is possible that with delayed gastric emptying, liquids are kept in the stomach too long, thereby causing biliary regurgitation. As a result of a stomach operation reflux from the duodenum or the small intestine to the stomach can increase. (Because after some operations the stomach no longer ends in the duodenum but rather in the jejunum, it is more appropriate to speak of enterogastric than duodenogastric reflux.) The following stomach operations result in enterogastric reflux (arranged in order of increasing severity):
— pyloroplasty
— truncal vagotomy with pyloroplasty
— gastrojejunostomy
— B-I gastrectomy
— B-II gastric resection
After the operation, biliary vomiting, epigastric complaints and nausea can develop. However it has not been established that pathological enterogastric reflux is a cause of gastritis, for gastritis can also be caused by postoperative gastric dymotility. Biliary vomiting can be treated with drugs that bind to bile salts (cholestyramin) or with motility-stimulating drugs. Severe biliary vomiting can be controlled by means of a Roux-en-Y operation.

Further examination

In a patient with upper abdominal symptoms it is important first to exclude organic causes. One can be dealing with anomalies outside the stomach (gall stones, pancreatitis, etc.) or organic anomalies of the stomach (tumour, ulcer, gastric outlet obstruction). The following methods of excluding organic anomalies are indicated: physical examination, blood analysis, endoscopy and ultrasonography (Intermezzo 13). Once organic disorders have been ruled out, a scintigraphic gastric emptying study is sometimes appropriate.

When to study gastric emptying?

In the following situations a gastric emptying study is necessary so that the optimal treatment can be chosen.
◆ Sometimes the doctor has doubts about whether slow or accelerated gastric emptying is involved; often the symptoms do not provide a basis for differentiating, and yet the treatment strategy in the two cases is different. A gastric emptying study is conclusive here.
◆ In a number of patients drug therapy is not effective. Sometimes a gastric emptying study can clarify why drug therapy has not been effective.
◆ In patients refractory to drug therapy who have severe symptoms, the

Intermezzo 13
Ruling out other disorders

Before gastric emptying and gastric motility are examined some obvious disorders should be ruled out.

◆ **Gastric and duodenal ulcer**
Generally there is a typical gnawing pain in the epigastrium that is relieved when the patient eats. With a duodenal ulcer there is often pain at night (hunger pangs). Diagnosis is made on the basis of endoscopy and possibly radiography.

◆ **Gastric carcinoma**. This disorder is to be suspected especially if there is loss of appetite and weight loss in the elderly patient and if the haemoglobin level is low. Diagnosis is made on the basis of endoscopy and a biopsy.

◆ **Gall stones**. Typical of this disorder are the postprandial colic attacks. The pain radiates mostly from the right costal margin around to the back. Diagnosis is made by means of ultrasonography or radiography.

◆ **Pancreatic carcinoma**. This disorder is to be suspected if there is a combination of weight loss (poor appetite) and pain in the upper abdomen and back in the older patient. As diagnostic aids first an ultrasonography is done and in some patients this is followed up by a CT-scan and endoscopic retrograde cholangiopancreaticography (ERCP, p. 283).

◆ Relapsing or chronic **pancreatitis**. Severe pain in the upper abdomen and back is often associated with this disorder. Diagnosis is based on a high serum- and urine-amylase determination, which is possibly followed up by a CT-scan and an ERCP.

◆ **Constipation**. This disorder is often associated with nagging upper abdominal pain attended by poor appetite and nausea. In the history taking the questioning should be focused on the frequency of defaecation and the consistency of the faeces. In examining the abdomen one will be able to feel faecal masses. A plain film of the abdomen can also contribute to the diagnosis.

doctor may wish to consider the possibility of a stomach operation. Such an operation is often irreversible. Before operating, one must therefore have the utmost confidence in the diagnosis.

◆ Sometimes after a stomach operation symptoms persist or new symptoms develop. In order to work out a strategy it is crucially important to gather data on gastric emptying.

Gastric emptying in different disorders

Upper abdominal symptoms in patients with diabetes mellitus can be caused by a delayed gastric emptying. A gastric emptying study can establish this aetiology. If diabetic gastroparesis is involved it is important to restore the gastric motility. A gastric emptying study is also a highly valuable aid in the investigation of postsurgical complaints. After a B-II operation or a truncal vagotomy with pyloroplasty the gastric emptying may have become too fast or too slow. On the basis of the gastric emptying study the doctor can rationally opt for reconstructive surgery. In some

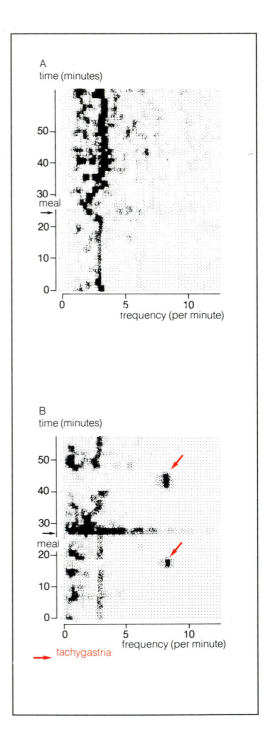

Figure 53: Frequency analysis of the electrogastrogram. A: Healthy volunteer. B: Patient with tachygastria. In this patient the frequency has transiently risen from 3 waves per minute to 9 waves per minute. During a tachygastric episode the stomach is quiescent. (Reproduced with permission, from Geldof, 1987). The term tachygastria is used only when the component consisting of 3 waves per minute, which coincides with the peristaltic contractions, is absent.

patients gastro-oesophageal reflux is a consequence of delayed gastric emptying. If a patient does not respond satisfactorily to anti-reflux therapy it can be useful to measure gastric emptying. It goes without saying that delayed gastric emptying is a contra-indication for anti-reflux surgery. An anti-reflux procedure can result in a minor vagal lesion, thereby further delaying gastric emptying. In patients with duodenal ulcers, gastric emptying is often accelerated but in some of them it is delayed. The delayed gastric emptying can be caused by a stenosis, but it can also be caused by a motility disturbance. If a highly selective vagotomy (HSV) is an option for a patient with recurrent duodenal ulcers, a gastric emptying study is important. If gastric emptying is delayed due to dysmotility, that is a contra-indication for an HSV.

In search of the cause of the disturbance

With the aid of gastric motility studies (manometry, EGG, ultrasonography) it is sometimes possible to identify the cause of the disordered gastric emptying. By means of an EGG, for example, a tachygastria can be shown immediately (Figure 53). During a tachygastria episode the frequency of the electrical control activity of the stomach increases (from 3 to as high as 9 depolarizations per minute or more) but the stomach no longer contracts. If the stomach is quiescent for too long, symptoms arise. Manometry can also directly demonstrate disordered gastric contractions (Figure 54). Through these studies the physiological basis of the disturbed gastric emptying can be revealed.

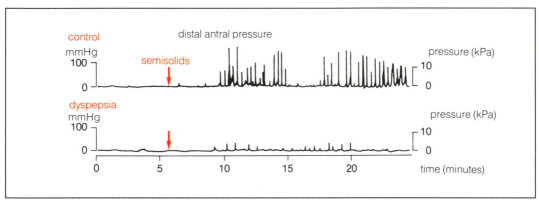

Figure 54: Manometric monitoring of the stomach after a meal in a healthy volunteer and a patient with dyspepsia. (Reproduced with permission, from Rees et al., 1980.)

Intermezzo 14
Definitions and concepts

The terms in which the patient's state (symptoms, syndrome, disorder, disease) can be expressed depend on the type of examination that has been performed (i.e. on the data available on the patient).

1. On the basis of **symptoms** one can make a diagnosis of dyspepsia. In this connection a number of symptoms are important:
— heartburn: points to gastro-oesophageal reflux
— early satiety: points to disturbed gastric emptying
— feeling of fullness: points to disturbed gastric emptying
— nausea and vomiting: points to disturbed gastric emptying
— retrosternal pain: can point to gastro-oesophageal reflux
— epigastric pain: can point to ulcer or disturbed gastric emptying
— vasomotor symptoms (the dumping syndrome): points to accelerated gastric emptying

2. On the basis of supplementary **endoscopic, ultrasonographic** or **radiographic** examination one can conclude:
— dyspepsia due to peptic ulceration
— dyspepsia with gastritis
— other organic disorders (tumour, stenosis)
— functional (non-ulcer) dyspepsia

3. On the basis of a **gastric emptying study** one can conclude:
— ......with delayed gastric emptying
— ......with accelerated gastric emptying
(The dotted lines can be filled in with a tentative diagnosis based on points 1 and 2; e.g. "functional dyspepsia with delayed gastric emptying".)

4. On the basis of a **motility study** (manometry, EGG, etc.) one can conclude:
— ......due to gastric dysrhythmias (amongst others, tachygastria)
— ......due to gastroparesis (of antrum or fundus)
— ......due to pyloric dysfunctions (excessive or insufficient resistance)
— ......due to disordered gastroduodenal co-ordination
(The dotted lines can be filled in with a tentative diagnosis based on points 1, 2 or 3; e.g. "functional dyspepsia caused by gastric dysrhythmias".)

Treatment

Drug therapy in delayed gastric emptying

For delayed gastric emptying due to gastric hypomotility prokinetics are the indicated drugs. A choice can be made from two classes of drugs (Chapter 14).

◆ Antagonists of the peripheral dopamine D_2-receptors: this group includes domperidone and metoclopramide.

◆ Drugs that stimulate the release of acetylcholine in the myenteric plexus: cisapride and to a lesser extent metoclopramide.

In contrast to metoclopramide, domperidone crosses the blood–brain barrier either not at all or only to a very slight extent and therefore has no extrapyramidal side-effects. Cisapride increases acetylcholine release only in the myenteric plexus and in this way promotes the contractions of the stomach and small intestine. All three prokinetics reinforce the motile co-ordination of antrum and proximal duodenum. Cisapride does this most markedly. It accelerates gastric emptying and controls symptoms in patients with idiopathic gastroparesis, anorexia nervosa, diabetic gastroparesis and postsurgical gastroparesis.

Surgical treatment of delayed gastric emptying

If drug therapy, possibly followed by dietary and lifestyle modifications, is not effective, an operation is sometimes the answer. After a gastric resection there are sometimes arguments in favour of a re-operation. Surgery deserves a cautious attitude, however, since an operation (or a re-operation) carries the risk of new motility disturbances.

Treatment of accelerated gastric emptying

Accelerated gastric emptying is much less prevalent than delayed gastric emptying. Until now, no drugs have been identified that are really useful in the treatment of accelerated gastric emptying. If patients have clearly defined symptoms and accelerated gastric emptying is established by means of a radio-isotopic method, the patient should be advised to eat frequent small meals, not to drink during the solid meal and to consume fewer carbohydrates. Consumption of a given class of food can control symptoms. For example, many fruits contain pectin, which can act as a binding agent, thereby somewhat delaying gastric emptying. Severe dumping symptoms are fortunately rare. If they are present, surgery is sometimes effective. A Roux-en-Y gastroenterostomy can be performed, which delays both gastric liquid and gastric solid emptying.

Conclusion

In the past 10 years we have acquired much knowledge about the motility of stomach, pylorus and proximal duodenum. It is known for example that gastric emptying is different for liquids and solids. Immediately after liquid has been ingested, the stomach begins to eliminate it. After a solid meal it takes several minutes for the stomach to grind, break down and hydrate the chyme to the point where it can be evacuated. Thus it takes 2–3 hours before most of the food is eliminated from the stomach. There is a control mechanism that ensures that the food reaches the duodenum in the proper amounts from the stomach. We have learned about this mechanism thanks to the development of better methods of investigation: radioisotopic techniques for investigating gastric emptying, intra-abdominal manometry and the EGG. The most important techniques are the non-invasive gastric emptying study with radio-labelled test meals and manometry of the stomach, pylorus and duodenum. With these techniques the effects of treatment can now be evaluated objectively. In addition, better and better drugs are being developed for the treatment of dysmotility of the stomach and duodenum. The most recent is cisapride. New pathophysiological insights allow us to judge if, and what type of, surgery is indicated. These developments have clearly increased the success of surgical treatment.

References

Geldof H. Electrogastrography: clinical applications. Rotterdam: Erasmus Universiteit. 1987

Read NW, Al-Jabani MN, Holgate AM, Barber DC, Edwards CA. Simultaneous measurement of gastric emptying, small bowel residence and colonic filling of a solid meal by the use of the gamma camera. Gut 1986; 27: 300–308

Rees WDW, Miller LJ, Malagelada JR. Dyspepsia, antral motor dysfunction, gastric stasis of solids. Gastroenterology 1980; 78: 360–365

Stacher G, e.a. Delayed gastric emptying in patients with anorexia nervosa and bulimia: effect of cisapride. Dig Dis Sci 1985; 30: 796

Chapter 8

The gallbladder and bile ducts

The transport of bile is carried out by the smooth muscle of the gallbladder and the sphincter of Oddi. Dysmotility of the gallbladder or the sphincter of Oddi can lead to the formation of gall stones, but also to typical pain attacks without gall stones. This type of pain was until recently not understood.

Introduction

The liver produces bile continuously, the amount easily reaching 800–1000 ml per day. Bile consists, amongst other substances, of water, bile salts, lecithin and cholesterol. It is secreted by the liver, transported through the bile ducts and stored in the gallbladder (Figure 55). During and after a meal the gallbladder empties the collected and concentrated bile into the duodenum. The bile salts are reabsorbed mainly in the last portion of the small intestine. They are absorbed by the liver for recycling. In this chapter we focus on the motility patterns of the gallbladder and bile ducts and the manner in which the bile is transported. In the past few years much information has come to light about the role of the motility of the gallbladder and the bile ducts in the genesis of a number of pathological conditions, like gall stone disease and dyskinesia of the sphincter of the bile ducts (the sphincter of Oddi).

Bile is necessary

Bile plays an important role in the digestion and absorption of fat and fat-soluble substances from the small intestine. If no bile reaches the small intestine little or no fat is absorbed. Bile is absent when the common bile duct is completely obstructed, and the clinical picture is then dominated by obstructive jaundice. Disordered fat absorption pales by comparison with this development. Severely disturbed fat resorption due to bile deficiency is in fact observed only in patients in whom the bile ducts have been percutaneously drained over a long

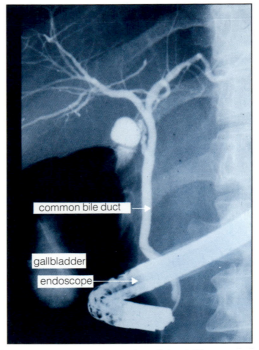

Figure 55: Radiography of the biliary tree by means of endoscopic retrograde cholangiopancreaticography (ERCP).

period. Disturbed fat absorption brings about steatorrhoea, weight loss and deficiencies in essential fatty acids and fat-soluble vitamins.

The gallbladder is not necessary

Although bile is necessary for the absorption of substances from the small intestine, the gallbladder is not indispensable. The function of the gallbladder is to concentrate the bile from the liver and to deliver it to the small intestine at the times at which it is needed. Delivery of the concentrated bile at the right times is not essential to good health however. This conclusion was reached on the basis of the following observations. First, it is sometimes appropriate to remove the gallbladder or to transect the sphincter of Oddi. These operations do not cause a noticeable disturbance of the fat balance. Second, there are animals that have no gallbladder (e.g. the rat).

Normal motility patterns of the biliary tract

The transport of bile is mainly controlled by three factors:
— bile production in the liver
— contractions of the gallbladder
—˙ contractions of the sphincter of Oddi.
The contractions of the gall bladder and sphincter of Oddi are different in the fasting state and the postprandial state (Figure 56).

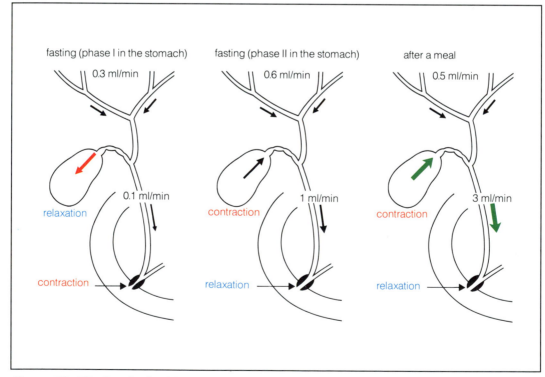

Figure 56: Bile flow in the biliary tree in the fasting and the postprandial state.

Intermezzo 15
Techniques for studying the motility of the biliary tract

Radiography
The **gallbladder** can be seen on radiographs that are made with an orally administered iodine-containing contrast medium. If radiographs are taken before and after contraction of the gallbladder one can get an idea of its contractile capacity. Contraction of the gallbladder can be stimulated by a fatty meal e.g. a standardized chocolate bar, or by intravenous administration of a diagnostic agent (CCK8 ["pancreozymin"] or ceruletide. The **bile ducts** can also be seen by means of radiography, in particular by endoscopic retrograde cholangiopancreaticography (ERCP, p. 283, Figure 55). With ERCP obstructions in the common bile duct and the pancreatic duct can be detected.

Ultrasonography
Ultrasonography is increasingly used as a substitute for radiography as a means of visualizing the gallbladder and, when they arise, gall stones, and of studying postprandial gallbladder emptying. By means of measurements in two directions, the volume of the gallbladder can be calculated (Figure 58). With this technique the (minor) interdigestive gallbladder emptying can also be observed.

HIDA scan
Bile transport can be observed with special radioactive tracers (the HIDA scan, p. 287). These tracers are selectively and efficiently filtered by the liver from the blood and excreted into the bile. Then transport of the bile can be followed with a gamma camera (as in gastric emptying studies).

Manometry of the sphincter of Oddi
By means of the instrumentation channel of a side-viewing fibrescope, a thin manometric catheter can be inserted into the papil of Vater and the common bile duct. The pressure in the biliary tract and the sphincter of Oddi can then be measured at several positions simultaneously if desired (p. 123, Figure 61).

The gallbladder

The gallbladder stores bile, concentrates it and excretes it at the appropriate time. The motility patterns of the gallbladder are co-ordinated with reference to these activities.

◆ **Postprandial**. After a meal and especially after a fatty meal there is a requirement for bile in the small intestine. At this point the gallbladder muscle contracts tonically, thereby evacuating part of its contents (Figure 57). The duration

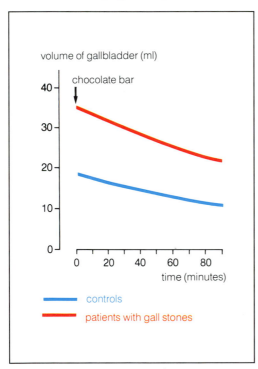

Figure 57: Postprandial gallbladder contractions elicited by a chocolate bar in healthy volunteers and patients with gall stones (measured by ultrasonography). (Reproduced with permission, from K.J. Van Erpecum, 1991.)

and force of the gallbladder contractions depend on the composition of the meal; if a meal contains a large quantity of fat, the gallbladder contracts with extra force and over a long interval. In healthy volunteers the average volume of the gallbladder is 20 ml. After they eat a chocolate bar about 10 ml of bile is excreted. Gallbladder emptying after a meal can be observed clearly by means of ultrasonography (Figure 58).

◆ **Interdigestive**. In the fasting state, most of the time the tonic pressure in the gallbladder is low (maximum: 0.3 kPa [2.5 mmHg]). Bile flows continuously into the gallbladder (0.5–1 ml/min). About 20% of the bile secreted by the liver flows directly to the duodenum. When stomach and duodenum enter phase II of the interdigestive migrating motor complex (MMC), the gallbladder wall contracts gradually (Figure 59), thereby expelling bile to the duodenum. In man this contraction lasts for dozens of minutes. At the end of phase II in the duodenum the gallbladder relaxes. The MMC is the mechanical and chemical "broom" of the gastrointestinal tract. The evacuation of the bile also contributes to this activity. After a meal more bile is eliminated than during phase II of the MMC.

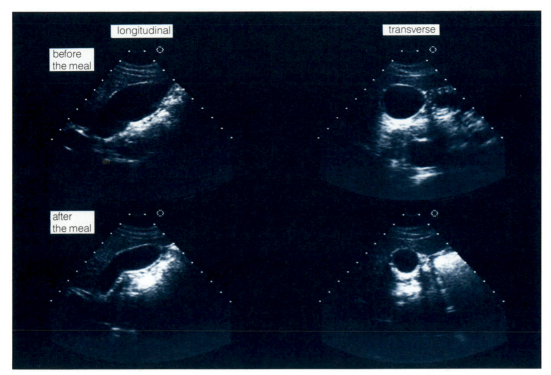

Figure 58: Ultrasonograms of the gallbladder before and after a meal. Measuring the volume of the gallbladder always requires recordings from two angles. (Reproduced with permission, from K.J. Van Erpecum.)

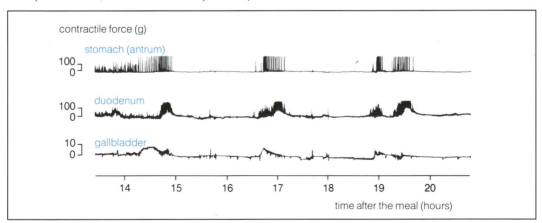

Figure 59: The gallbladder wall contracts when the MMC in the stomach is in phase II (measured by means of strain gauges). These data cannot be converted directly into intra-gallbladder pressures. (Reproduced with permission, from Itoh, 1983.)

The sphincter of Oddi

After a meal the sphincter of Oddi opens and bile can flow easily to the duodenum. In the fasting state the movements of the sphincter of Oddi are more complex, involving tonic and phasic contractions.

◆ **Tonic contractions**. The sphincter of Oddi is constricted much of the time. The resting pressure is 1.3–3 kPa (10–25 mmHg), which is about 1 kPa higher than the pressure in the common bile and pancreatic ducts. A contracted sphincter of Oddi contributes to bile flow into the gallbladder*.

◆ **Phasic contractions**. The basis of the phasic contractions of the sphincter of Oddi is the depolarization of the smooth muscle

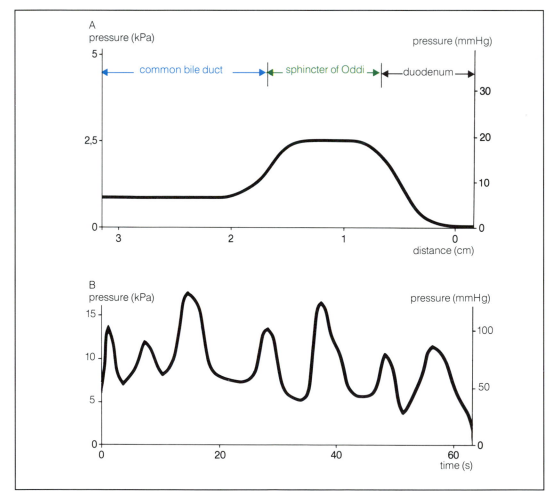

Figure 60: Pressure in the sphincter of Oddi. A: Average pull-through profile. B: Measurement with stationary pressure sensor: phasic contractions can be seen.

* Not all the factors in this process are understood. If the sphincter of Oddi of patients is transected, the bile still flows into the gallbladder. How this happens is not known. At the juncture between the gallbladder and the cystic duct there is a fold that might function as a kind of valve.

cells. These continuously produce a regular pattern of depolarization and hyperpolarization, i.e. the electrical control activity (ECA, p. 42), like the one observed in the stomach and duodenum. In the sphincter of Oddi the frequency of the electrical control activity is about 12 depolarizations per minute (the same as in the duodenum). The depolarizations determine the times at which spike bursts (see p. 43: electrical response activity, ERA) can occur, which are accompanied by phasic contractions. The frequency of these is about 4 waves per minute and the waves have an amplitude of 17 kPa (130 mmHg, Figure 60). These phasic contractions are generally propagated toward the duodenum (antegrade, Figure 61), but

retrograde (13%) and simultaneous contractions (26%) also occur. There is evidence that phasic activity is at least as important in regulating the bile flow as tonic activity. The antegrade phasic contractions of the sphincter of Oddi milk the common bile duct dry as it were. The sphincter of Oddi is not a secure barrier: even in the fasting state a small quantity of bile leaks out to the duodenum.

The common bile duct

The wall of the common bile duct contains scarcely any smooth muscle and therefore manifests little motor activity. There are, however, limited pressure fluctuations in the lumen of the common bile duct but these are probably caused by the contractions of the gallbladder and the sphincter of Oddi.

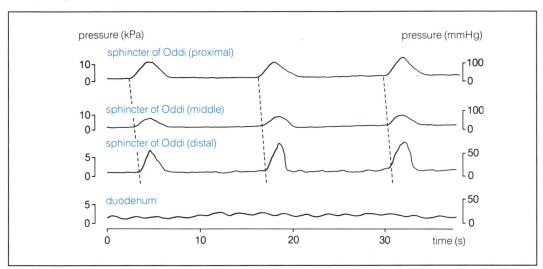

Figure 61: Normal contractions of the sphincter of Oddi in man, recorded with three intraluminal pressure sensors positioned at intervals of 2 mm. The intraduodenal pressure was measured with a separate catheter. (Reproduced with permission, from Hogan et al., 1983.)

Control of motility of the biliary tract

Neuronal influence

The biliary system is subject to neuronal and hormonal regulation. More is known about the hormonal control. The gallbladder and bile ducts are parasympathetically innervated by a branch of the vagal nerve. The sympathetic fibres reach the region from the coeliac ganglion. A mucosal and myenteric plexus are found in the wall of the gallbladder itself. There is a high concentration of nerve cells in the wall of the bile duct but these do not form a well-defined intramural plexus. In the sphincter of Oddi on the other hand there is a dense network of nerve cells. The role of the parasympathetic innervation becomes clear after vagotomy: the gallbladder is relaxed and dilated. It is assumed that the vagal nerve also stimulates the contractions of the sphincter of Oddi. It has been established, for example, that cholinergic agents stimulate contractions of the sphincter and anticholinergic agents inhibit them (see Table 5, p. 127). However, even after denervation the sphincter maintains its basal pressure and phasic contractions persist. It is believed that the biliary tract is affected by different neurotransmitters but this regulation has been little investigated to date. There are however classes of drugs that raise or lower the basal pressure of the sphincter of Oddi. For the moment though it is not clear whether these drugs are effective in controlling dysmotility of the biliary system.

Hormonal influence

We shall mention here two hormones that have a pronounced effect on the biliary system: motilin and cholecystokinin.

◆ **Motilin** is a peptide produced in the cells of the proximal small intestine. This hormone is of particular significance to the gastrointestinal tract since its concentration in the plasma rises when phase II of the MMC starts in the stomach (Figure 62). During phase III in the stomach the concentration of motilin in the blood is maximal. The concentration of motilin in the plasma also shows a clear relationship with the gallbladder contractions. Does plasmatic motilin induce the gallbladder contractions or

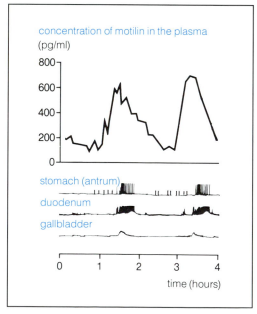

Figure 62: When the MMC in the stomach and duodenum is in phase III, the concentration of endogenous motilin rises in the blood. (Reproduced with permission, from Itoh et al., 1983.)

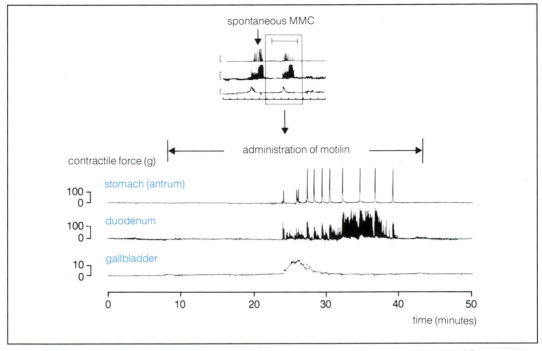

spontaneous MMC

administration of motilin

contractile force (g)

stomach (antrum)

duodenum

gallbladder

0   10   20   30   40   50

time (minutes)

Figure 63: After administration of synthetic motilin, phases II and III of the MMC start in the stomach and duodenum (prematurely) and the gallbladder contracts. (Reproduced with permission, from Itoh et al., 1983.)

does duodenal bile cause the release of motilin? Some researchers suspect that duodenal bile stimulates the release of motilin; it is shown that the peak plasma level of motilin is reached only after the gallbladder has contracted. Other workers believe that the motilin in the blood causes the gallbladder to contract, so that simultaneously phase II of the MMC (and immediately thereafter phase III) is activated in the stomach and the duodenum.

◆ **Cholecystokinin** (CCK) is a peptide that is made and secreted by cells in the duodenum and jejunum. It is secreted as a peptide consisting of 33 amino acids (CCK33) or as a fragment consisting of 8 amino acids (CCK8). Both substances are biologically active. CCK is released as a reaction to fatty compounds in the small intestine. It elicits contraction of the gallbladder and relaxation of the sphincter of Oddi. It is likely that CCK is the most important factor in post-prandial relaxation of the sphincter of Oddi. By the simultaneous contraction of the gallbladder and relaxation of the sphincter of Oddi, a large quantity of bile is transported to the duodenum. CCK is thus an important step in the process underlying the promotion of fat absorption.

Motility disorders of the biliary tract

Disorders of the biliary tract automatically suggest gall stones. We shall see however that many persons have gall stones without the associated symptoms and many patients have "gall stone symptoms" without a gall stone.

Symptoms of gall stones
The classical pain with gall stones is located in the right upper abdomen and it often radiates to the right, around to the back. Often this pain is accompanied by nausea and vomiting. This symptom generally occurs after a meal. Very typical but relatively rare is biliary colic, characterized by severe pain.

Gall stones
In the gallbladder the bile is concentrated. However, if the bile is supersaturated, crystals form from its constituents. The term gall stone is used when larger concretions of crystals and calcium, etc., form (Figure 64). In Western Europe a high percentage of the population has gall stones; a prevalence study has revealed that about 7% of men and 15% of women have demonstrable gall stones. Only a small proportion of these persons have the associated symptoms. Cholesterol gall stones are mostly involved. This type of stone is provoked by the following factors:
— insufficient secretion of bile acids
— excessive secretion of cholesterol
— deficient gallbladder emptying.
It is generally held that gall stones, either whole or in pieces, are particularly apt to produce symptoms when they reach the common bile duct.

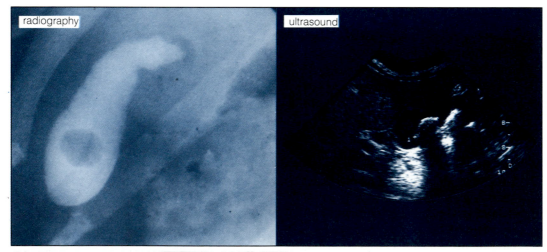

radiography

ultrasound

Figure 64: Radiographic and ultrasonographic images of the same gallbladder with a gall stone. Typical of the ultrasonographic image is the acoustic shadow behind the stone. (Reproduced with permission, from M.F.J. Stolk.)

Gallbladder motility and the formation of gall stones

Patients with gall stones generally have disordered gallbladder emptying. The volume of their gallbladder, especially in the fasting state, is much greater than that of controls (Figure 57). What is the cause of these disturbances and what are its consequences?

— Gall stones can impede gallbladder emptying.
— Also the bile in the gallbladder can become supersaturated as a result of insufficient emptying, so that gall stones form.

It is believed that in at least a certain number of patients insufficient emptying of the gallbladder caused gall stones to form. It is likely that a decrease of both the postprandial and the interdigestive gallbladder emptying contributes to the formation, but only the postprandial emptying is easy to study. Delayed gallbladder emptying is found in the following groups at risk from gall stones: pregnant women and patients on total parenteral nutrition, mellitus patients, patients having post-vagotomy status or somatostatinoma. Already before the formation of gall stones, in a portion of the persons belonging to these risk groups, there is diminished gallbladder emptying. In the others, however, gallbladder emptying is normal. Similarly, the results of animal studies indicate that disturbed gallbladder emptying is often a cause rather than a consequence of gall stones.

Dyskinesia of the sphincter of Oddi

The same symptoms as those associated with gall stones are observed when the passage through the sphincter of Oddi is impeded. The impediment can arise from an organic stenosis (sclerosis, fibrosis or tumour) or an abnormal motility (dyskinesia). In recent years it has been established that dyskinesia of the sphincter of Oddi constitutes a real pathological profile. Motility disorders of the sphincter of Oddi are found in different conditions:

— other diseases such as systemic sclerosis, diabetes mellitus or chronic idiopathic intestinal pseudo-obstruction (CIIP)
— drug-induced conditions (Table 5); the biliary tract is extremely sensitive to opiates: pain due to biliary tract disorders is not eliminated by opiates; on the contrary, it is exacerbated.
— conditions of unknown origin (idiopathic).

It is now known that not only gall stones, but every stimulus or stretch of the gallbladder or bile ducts can bring on the symptoms that appear to be so typical of gall stones.

---

increasing sphincter tone:
— cholinergic agonists
— α-agonists
— H_1-agonists
— opiates

decreasing sphincter tone:
— β-agonists
— muscarinic blockers (anticholinergic agents)
— calcium antagonists
— nitrates

Table 5: Classes of drugs thought to affect gallbladder pressure.

Dyskinesia of the sphincter of Oddi is most prevalent in patients whose gallbladder has been previously resected. The interpretation of this finding is unclear. Does resection of the gallbladder lead secondarily to disorders of the sphincter of Oddi? Or is resection of the gallbladder in these patients not such a wise operation? Would it perhaps not be better to cut the sphincter of Oddi (Intermezzo 16)?

Dyskinesia of the sphincter of Oddi: diagnosis and treatment

The diagnosis "dyskinesia of the sphincter of Oddi" was put on an objective footing only a short while ago, thanks to the arrival of advanced study techniques. Based on the symptom pattern, as a rule one examines these patients first for gall stones. These are not found in these patients but there are signs in the blood of obstruction of the bile ducts. These signs include a transient rise in the enzymes alkaline phosphatase and gamma-glutamyltransferase (γ-GT). By means of endoscopic retrograde cholangiopancreaticography (ERCP) it can often be established that the common bile duct is slightly dilated. But when the patient presents no biochemical nor morphological anomalies, diagnosis is difficult. In that case pressure measurements in the sphincter of Oddi is the only way of substantiating a diagnosis. Manometry reveals an elevated basal sphincter pressure (above 5 kPa [40 mmHg]) in a number of patients. This condition is described as dyskinesia of the sphincter of Oddi, although it would be more precise if the label were "achalasia of the sphincter of Oddi".

In addition, there is a higher proportion of retrograde phasic contractions in the sphincter of these patients. In some, the frequency of the phasic contractions is high ("tachyoddia"). If the diagnosis of dyskinesia of the sphincter of Oddi is supported by manometric findings, endoscopic sphincterotomy can be useful. In this procedure the sphincter of Oddi is transected with a metal wire and a diathermal current. Then, the common bile duct is no longer obstructed. It has not yet been properly investigated whether drugs can repair dyskinesia of the sphincter of Oddi. However, it is established that the following drugs relax smooth muscle:
— nitrates: nitroglycerin isosorbide dinitrate or pentaeritrityl tetranitrate
— calcium antagonists: nifedipine or diltiazem

If the pressure in the sphincter of Oddi is not high, it can be very difficult to make a diagnosis and decide on a treatment; certainly a sphincterotomy is not useful.

Intermezzo 16
Case study: a patient with dyskinesia of the sphincter of Oddi

The patient is a 43-year-old woman who had previously had a cholecystectomy. This was done because she had had frequent colic attacks in the right upper abdomen that radiated to the back. A radiographic examination and ultrasonography of the gallbladder disclosed that she had multiple small gall stones. She withstood the operation without problems but a few months later the colic attacks recurred. The attacks occurred irregularly but mostly in the evening or early at night. Twice, each time early in the morning after an attack, blood was taken for analysis. A slight elevation of alkaline phosphatase and γ-GT was found. An ultrasonographic study was negative: the bile ducts were not dilated. An ERCP was performed, which showed a slightly dilated common bile duct with normal intrahepatic bile ducts. The pancreatic duct was normal. It was decided to perform manometry of the sphincter of Oddi and the basal pressure in the sphincter of Oddi was measured at 7 kPa (53 mmHg). The phasic contractions had a maximum frequency of 4 waves per minute. Tachyoddia was thus excluded. It was a plausible hypothesis that the symptoms were induced by a high basal pressure of the sphincter of Oddi. It was then decided to do an endoscopic sphincterotomy. This was performed one year after the cholecystectomy. Two years have now passed since this procedure and the patient is almost symptom-free. From time to time she still has pain attacks in the right upper abdomen but these do not require further treatment.

Conclusion

Often symptoms involving the gallbladder and bile ducts are caused by gall stones. These stones sometimes form because gallbladder emptying is delayed. However, some patients with the typical "gall stone pain" don't have gall stones. Thanks to new study techniques (in particular ultrasonography and manometry of the sphincter of Oddi) it is frequently possible to identify motility disturbances of the gallbladder or the sphincter of Oddi. The typical symptoms of gallstones can also arise from motility disturbances of the biliary tract. An endoscopic intervention can now be performed when the pressure in the sphincter of Oddi is elevated.

References

Dodds WJ, Hogan WJ, Geenen JE. Perspectives about function of the sphincter of Oddi. Viewpoint Dig Dis 1988; 20: 9–12

Erpecum KJ van, Berge Henegouwen GP van. Pathogenic factors in cholesterol gallstone disease. Scand J Gastroenterol 1989; 24: S171: 81–90.

Fullarton GM, Hilditch T, Campbell A, Murray WR. Clinical and scintigraphic assessment of the role of endoscopic sphincterectomy in the treatment of sphincter of Oddi dysfunction. Gut 1990; 31: 231–235

Hogan WJ, e.a. Motility and biliary dyskinesia. In: Chey WY, ed. Functional disorders of the digestive tract. New York: Raven Press 1983: 267–275

Itoh Z, Takahashi I, Nakaya M, Suzuki T. Interdigestive function of the gallbladder of the dog. In: Chey WY, ed. Functional disorders of the digestive tract. New York: Raven Press 1983: 259–265

Pomeranz IS, Shaffer EAA. Abnormal gallbladder emptying in a subgroup of patients with gallstones. Gastroenterology 1985; 88: 787–791

The small intestine

Disorders of the motility patterns of the small intestine are difficult to identify, but it is assumed that they are not rare. It is likely that they contribute to a variety of upper and lower abdominal complaints that are as yet not understood. Severe motility disorders of the small intestine can be life-threatening.

Introduction

Upper and lower abdominal complaints are sometimes associated with a motility disturbance of the stomach or colon, but may also be caused by dysmotility of the small intestine. The problem with the small intestine is that little is known about its movements because this organ, owing to its position and its many twisting loops, is much harder to examine than the stomach or large intestine. Until recently the most important information about the motility of the small intestine was obtained by means of radiographic examination. Now other methods for studying this activity have been developed. The small intestine transit time for chyme can be measured by means of the breath hydrogen test (p. 290) or scintigraphy (p. 286). With the aid of manometry the contractions of segments of the small intestine can be measured.

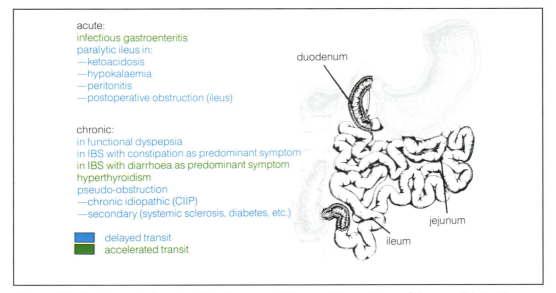

acute:
infectious gastroenteritis
paralytic ileus in:
—ketoacidosis
—hypokalaemia
—peritonitis
—postoperative obstruction (ileus)

chronic:
in functional dyspepsia
in IBS with constipation as predominant symptom
in IBS with diarrhoea as predominant symptom
hyperthyroidism
pseudo-obstruction
—chronic idiopathic (CIIP)
—secondary (systemic sclerosis, diabetes, etc.)

■ delayed transit
■ accelerated transit

duodenum

jejunum

ileum

Figure 65: Acute and chronic disturbances of the motility pattern of the small intestine.

Normal movements of the small intestine

The smooth muscle cells of the small intestine

The smooth muscle cells of the small intestine produce a regular electrical control activity. In man the frequency of the electrical control activity of the duodenum is about 12 depolarizations per minute. From the duodenum to the ileum there is a gradual decrease in frequency to about 8 depolarizations per minute. Only if this depolarization is accompanied by action potentials does the smooth muscle contract.

Motor patterns

Not only in the stomach but also in the small intestine is the motility pattern after a meal different from that in the fasting state.

♦ After a meal the contents of the small intestine are slowly transported distally, in the food absorption phase. At that point fairly irregular phasic contractions are initiated in the small intestine, which are propagated over only a short intestinal segment (Figure 66). The number and the force of the contractions depend on the composition of the food. The number of contractions or action potentials after a meal containing a large quantity of glucose is for instance greater than after a meal containing a large quantity of fat.

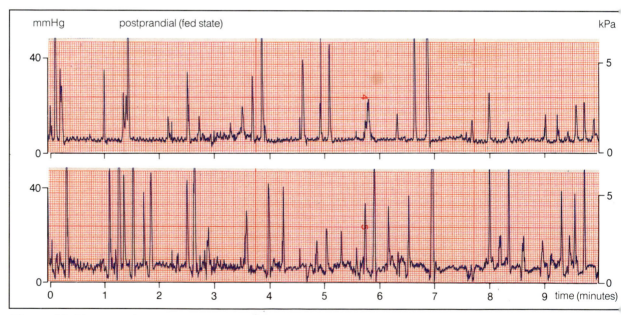

Figure 66: Manometric monitoring of the small intestine. (Recordings were made at 5 cm intervals.) The postprandial pattern is characterized by irregular contractions with a relatively low amplitude.

◆ In the interdigestive state the small intestine is almost empty. The MMC also occurs in the small intestine (Figure 67). This activity pattern generally begins in the stomach but can also begin in the small intestine. It travels slowly (5–10 cm per minute) toward the ileum. Often it does not reach the terminal ileum, dying out more proximally in the small intestine.

Transport through the small intestine

The pattern of transport in the small intestine is also completely different postprandially and during the interdigestive state.

◆ **Interdigestive**. When the stomach is (almost) empty, the postprandial pattern is followed by the MMC. Indigestible solid food particles leave the stomach during phase III of the MMC. Together with cellular debris they are transported to the terminal ileum in about 1.5 hours under the control of the MMC. The most important function of the MMC is to prevent stasis of the small intestine, thereby also preventing bacterial overgrowth.

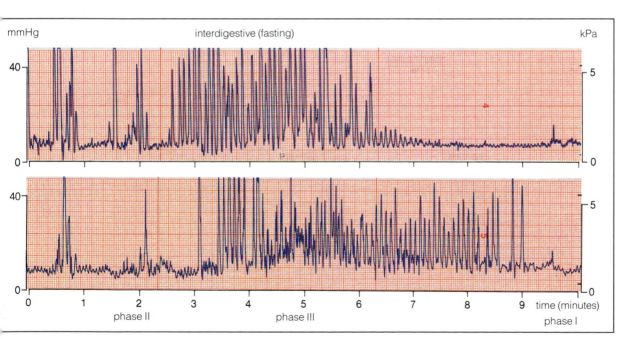

Figure 67: The interdigestive pattern: during phase III there are strong contractions at the maximum frequency.

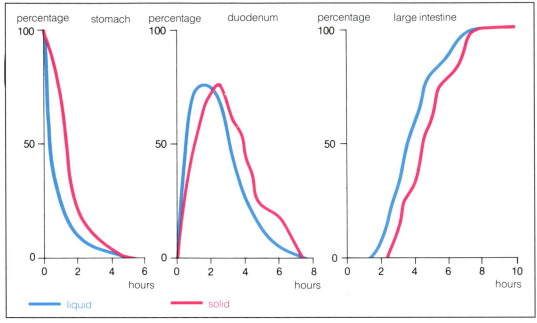

Figure 68: Passage of a liquid or solid meal from the stomach along the small intestine to the colon, measured by scintigraphy in a healthy volunteer. (Data on solid meal reproduced with permission, from Read et al., 1986.)

◆ **Postprandial**. Figure 68 shows the passage of the food through the stomach and the small intestine. There is a control system that ensures that the stomach delivers to the small intestine finely regulated quantities of chyme with a fairly constant consistency and composition (p. 98). Once the chyme from the stomach reaches the duodenum, the transit rate is the same whether the meal was solid or liquid.

Factors affecting transport through the small intestine

Whilst the **consistency** of the meal (solid, semisolid or liquid) significantly affects gastric emptying, this factor has almost no influence on small intestinal transit time. On the other hand, the **composition** of the chyme in the small intestine does have an effect on transit. Fat in the food delays transit. When (non-absorbed) fat reaches the last portion of the ileum, a reflex-controlled inhibition of gastric emptying—the ileal brake—is activated. **Psychic stress** can accelerate transit through the small intestine, whilst **physical effort** delays it. These effects come about via the vagal nerve and the sympathetic system.

Symptoms and physical examination

Disorders of the small intestine seldom result in a characteristic pattern of symptoms. The symptoms more or less mimic those provoked by gastric emptying disorders: feeling of fullness, nausea, vomiting, cramps, pain and abdominal distension after a meal. In addition diarrhoea and weight loss can occur. Suggestions for a diagnostic examination of patients with these symptoms are given on pp. 218–222. A fairly typical symptom pattern is associated with obstruction ileus and paralytic ileus. In both there is severe pain and abdominal distension. In paralytic ileus the pain is more or less constant, whereas in obstruction ileus it is often intermittent. In obstruction ileus, on auscultation one finds loud noises of high frequency; often one also hears "high-pitched bowel sounds". In paralytic ileus, on auscultation one finds no or almost no noise. Unfortunately there is no symptom that could be used to differentiate with certainty organic from non-organic anomalies. For this differentiation further examination is necessary (p. 222).

The disorders

Disorders of the movements of the small intestine can occur in acute or chronic form. With infections of the gastrointestinal tract (gastroenteritis) small intestinal transit is accelerated. Together with an increase in water secretion this development produces diarrhoea. Chronic symptoms often pose a greater problem for diagnosis and treatment than acute symptoms.

Obstruction ileus and paralytic ileus

Ileus is a frequently occurring acute disorder of the small intestinal transit. A distinction is made between two main types of ileus: obstruction and paralytic ileus.

◆ In **obstruction ileus** the intestinal lumen is narrowed or closed. Passage is impeded but the small intestine still "tries" to transport its contents past the blockage. This effort brings about strong intestinal contractions.

◆ In **paralytic ileus** the contractions of the small intestine are diminished or absent. Often the cause of a paralytic ileus is easy to identify: for instance the sequelae of a major intra-abdominal operation (post-operative ileus), intra-abdominal infections (peritonitis, abscess) or a severe metabolic dysregulation (diabetic ketoacidosis, hypokalaemia). The treatment of paralytic ileus should therefore consist in eliminating the underlying cause.

Both forms of ileus are accompanied by severe pain and abdominal distension. In both a plain film of the standing patient reveals dilated bowel loops with air fluid levels. Generally, obstruction ileus can be clearly differentiated from paralytic ileus by means of auscultation. In both cases there is a risk of perforation of the intestinal wall and insufficient circulation, resulting in necrosis. Both complications are life-threatening. If an obstruction ileus is suspected, therefore, it should be decided rapidly to perform an exploratory laparotomy With the abdomen opened, the surgeon can determine the cause of the ileus and on the basis of his findings carry out other actions.

Functional dyspepsia: stomach and small intestine

Functional dyspepsia was discussed in Chapter 7. In a routine examination of dyspepsia no abnormalities are found. Yet gastric emptying, especially of solid food, is delayed. Manometric examination often discloses that the antrum produces contractions of insufficient frequency and strength after a meal. In some patients this also occurs

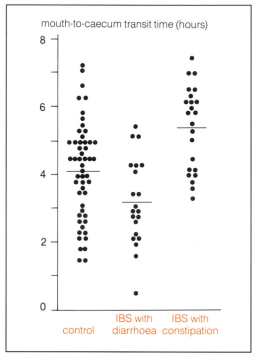

Figure 70: Mouth-to-colon transit time in healthy volunteers, IBS patients with diarrhoea and IBS patients with constipation. (Reproduced with permission, from Cann et al., 1987.)

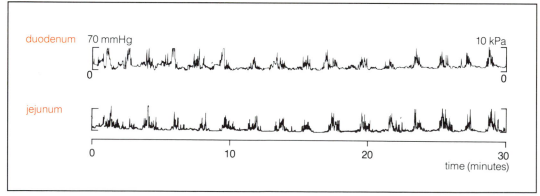

Figure 69: Intraluminal pressure measurement in the jejunum of a patient with IBS; abnormal, grouped contractions are clearly visible. (Reproduced with permission, from Kellow and Phillips, 1983.)

in the proximal part of the small intestine, again after a meal. In addition, the MMC is often disturbed in the small intestine. Dysmotility is therefore not limited to the stomach. This condition is referred to as "gastroduodenal motor dysfunction".

IBS: large and small intestine

IBS is above all a disturbance of the large intestine (see Chapter 10). However, in some patients with IBS, motility of the small intestine is also disturbed. They show an irregular MMC, some even showing no MMC at all, especially under stress. When the patient has abdominal pain, manometry often reveals groups of strong contractions of the small intestine (Figure 69). Small intestine transit time is also abnormal in some patients. In IBS patients in whom diarrhoea is the main symptom mean transit time is short, and in IBS patients in whom constipation is the main symptom it is prolonged (Figure 70).

Intermezzo 17
Examination of the small intestine

◆ **Radiographic examination** (with or without barium contrast) and **endoscopy** are indispensable in diagnosing intestinal symptoms, since with these techniques organic anomalies can be shown. With a flexible endoscope it is also possible to reach the most proximal and the most distal part of the small intestine, i.e. the duodenum and the terminal ileum. These methods or **laparotomy** make it possible to exclude structural anomalies and consider the possibility of motility disorders of the small intestine. These disorders are not disclosed by radiographic and endoscopic examination. In contrast, with the breath hydrogen test or scintigraphy, transport through the small intestine can be measured and with manometry, pressure variations can be measured.

◆ With the **breath hydrogen test** (Figure 131, p. 290) the mouth-to-caecum transit time can be determined.

◆ **Scintigraphic** examination of the small intestine is conducted in the same way as in the stomach (p. 286, cf. Figure 68). The time point at which the first radioactive material reaches the caecum is generally an appropriate parameter to determine. Abnormal transit through the small intestine can be determined more accurately by scintigraphy than by a radiographic examination. Also, the effect of drugs on small intestine transit can be better evaluated by scintigraphy.

◆ For a **manometric** study of the small intestine a perfused catheter is generally used. It is passed through the pylorus under X-ray control.

Chronic intestinal pseudo-obstruction (CIP)

Some patients present with the symptoms of an obstruction ileus *and* the signs thereof at the physical examination (abdominal distension, ileus-peristalsis). In addition, in some patients passage through the stomach or large intestine is impeded. At laparotomy, however, no sign of an obstruction is apparent, although the small intestine or a part of it is dilated. This profile is described as "pseudo-obstruction". This type of pseudo-obstruction is in fact a motility disorder. It can occur at any age and often takes a chronic intermittent course, in which case the label chronic intestinal pseudo-obstruction (CIP) is applied. It is often impossible to differentiate an organic obstruction from a pseudo-obstruction on the basis of a physical examination. Only an exploratory laparotomy is conclusive, however. Some forms of CIP are secondary to another often diagnosed earlier disorder like systemic sclerosis, diabetes mellitus, amyloidosis, radiation enteritis, lead poisoning or Chagas' disease (an infection known in South America and caused by *Trypanosoma cruzi*). In some patients CIP is caused by a tumour at another site in the body (paraneoplastic). In other patients with CIP no cause can be found. These are the so-called idiopathic forms.

Chronic idiopathic intestinal pseudo-obstruction (CIIP)

If in a patient with CIP no motility-related disorder can be found, the term chronic idiopathic intestinal pseudo-obstruction is used (p. 243). At present two forms of CIIP are distinguished:

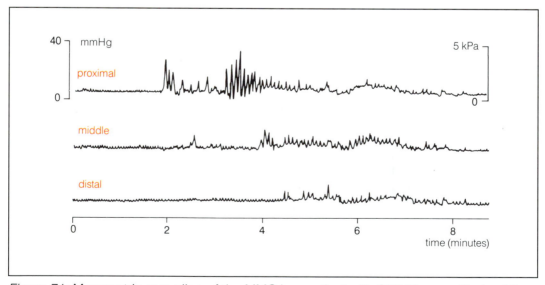

Figure 71: Manometric recording of the MMC in a patient with CIIP. The amplitude of the contractions is diminished.

◆ A disorder of the smooth muscle: myopathy (hollow visceral myopathy). In this disease other organs containing smooth muscle (e.g. the ureters, bladder and urethra) are often affected.

◆ A disorder of the nerve cells of the gastrointestinal tract: intestinal neuropathy. This disease can be accompanied by other neurological abnormalities.

Both forms of CIIP were discovered through microscopic examination of biopsies containing all the layers of the intestinal wall. In addition to biopsy **only manometry** is suitable for differentiating the two forms. In intestinal neuropathy the contractions are unco-ordinated but their amplitude is normal. In myopathy the converse is true: the contractions are reasonably co-ordinated but their force is diminished (Figure 71). The two forms cannot be distinguished radiologically. On a plain film of the abdomen dilated small bowel loops can be seen during an exacerbation, generally most clearly in the duodenum (Figure 72). Nor can the two forms of CIIP be distinguished by means of a barium contrast study of the small intestine. Moreover, the image with secondary CIP (e.g. in systemic sclerosis) often cannot be differentiated from that with CIIP (Figure 73). Nor are the breath hydrogen test and scintigraphy suitable for detecting myopathy and neuropathy in the small intestine. Clinically, patients with CIIP present with signs of intermittent ileus. Because an effective MMC is absent, stasis occurs in the small intestine, resulting in bacterial overgrowth.

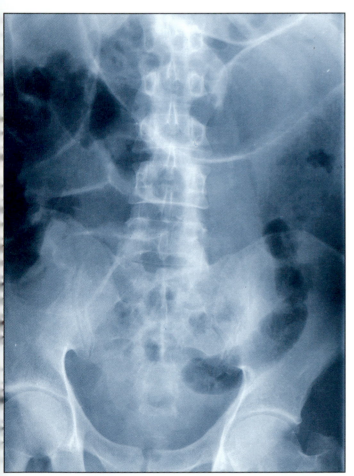

Figure 72: Abdominal overview of a patient with CIIP. The small bowel loops are clearly dilated.

The examination

Often further examination is desirable in patients in whom disorders of the small intestine are suspected.

- ◆ If the symptoms are fairly mild and present a pattern suggesting dyspepsia or IBS, generally a trial treatment is started. Only if the symptoms are severe or not controlled by treatment should one proceed to further examination.
- ◆ If there are acute intermittent or chronic symptoms as in ileus, first, **plain films of the abdomen** should be taken: if the patient is lying down, dilated intestinal loops can be seen in detail; if he or she is standing, air fluid levels in the intestines can be seen.
- ◆ If the physical examination gives indications of paralytic ileus, there should first be an attempt to identify the cause of what is observed.
- ◆ When there is strong evidence of an obstruction ileus (on the basis of the physical examination or the plain film of the abdomen), a **laparotomy** should be performed without delay. This procedure will make it possible to find the cause of the obstruction.
- ◆ If the signs of ileus are not pronounced a **barium-contrast radiographic examination** of the small intestine is recommended. In this way a partial obstruction can be detected. If the signs of ileus disappear spontaneously, it is likely that they will recur. It is therefore important to track down the cause of these signs with a barium-contrast radiographic examination.

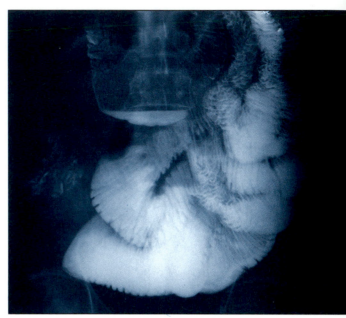

Figure 73: Radiograph of the small intestine in a patient with CIIP.

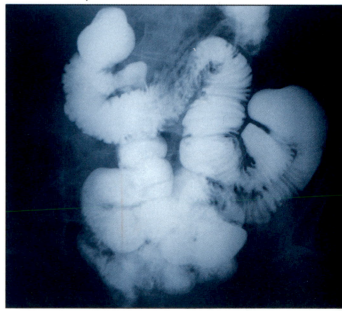

Figure 74: Radiograph of the small intestine in a patient with systemic sclerosis.

◆ Symptoms and signs consistent with an obstruction can also be caused by a "pseudo-obstruction". To investigate this possibility one can determine the intestinal transit time by means of the **breath hydrogen test and scintigraphy**. In patients with pseudo-obstruction (CIP or CIIP) bacterial overgrowth of the small intestine is always involved. These bacteria produce hydrogen, which can cause an early (or normal) peak in the breath hydrogen curve, even when transit time is decreased. Combining the breath hydrogen test with scintigraphy can be effective in differentiating a delayed from a normal passage.

◆ **Manometry** is suitable for further investigating the cause of the abnormality in pseudo-obstruction. In this way it can be determined whether a myopathy or a neuropathy is primarily involved.

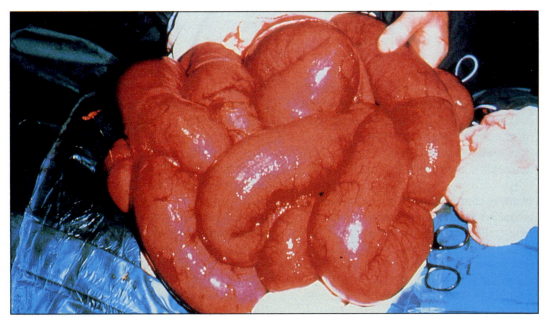

Figure 75: CIIP is characterized by severely dilated intestinal loops with bacterial overgrowth.

The treatment

Secondary motility disturbances of the small intestine

In secondary forms of dysmotility of the small intestine (such as in **infections** of the gastrointestinal tract and **metabolic dysregulation**) treatment of the primary disease process is crucial. The stomach and small intestine must not be unnecessarily stressed. For this reason it is sometimes appropriate to withold food from the patient. In addition, a gastric tube can be helpful so that the 1.5 litres of gastric juice produced by the stomach per day can be drained off.

The treatment of ileus

In **paralytic ileus** one should attempt to correct the underlying causal factor. Often a laparotomy is necessary for the diagnosis; if an intra-abdominal abscess is found, it can be immediately remedied. Or if laparotomy turns up an **obstruction ileus**, immediate surgical repair is necessary. If obstruction ileus or paralytic ileus is present, the patient must not be fed through the stomach, but intravenously. In addition, it is often necessary to drain off the gastric juice.

Motility disturbances of the small intestine in functional dyspepsia

In functional dyspepsia with a disordered small intestine one should first attempt to repair the dysmotility of the small intestine. Cholinesterase inhibitors, owing to their numerous side-effects, are seldom used. Dopamine-receptor blockade with domperidone is not particularly effective in promoting motility of the small intestine. More effective are drugs that stimulate release of acetylcholine in the myenteric plexus—in particular cisapride and to a lesser extent metoclopramide.

Motility disturbances of the small intestine in IBS

For patients with IBS accompanied by disorders of the small intestine, fibre-rich food should be prescribed before any other measure is taken. Theoretically, prokinetics that release acetylcholine would be expected to be of use to IBS patients whose predominant symptom is constipation. These drugs of course stimulate intestinal motility and therefore should afford a means of combatting the constipation.

Treatment of CIP and CIIP

In **secondary forms** of CIP, treatment of the primary disorder should be attempted. With (**primary**) **CIIP** this is not possible. With severe ileus symptoms, complete fasting, gastric drainage and intravenous fluid administration are necessary. In some patients continuous administration of food through a gastric tube is effective in reducing symptom severity. With chronic forms, gastrointestinal motility can be stimulated with prokinetics that release acetylcholine. Part of the problem arises from bacterial overgrowth, which often necessitates treatment with antibiotics. Drugs that decrease intestinal motility should of course be avoided. If possible the drugs of particular concern in this connection are those having anticholinergic (side-)effects and opiates. Some patients with CIIP are not capable in the long term of absorbing sufficient food via the gastrointestinal tract. They should therefore be put on a chronic parenteral nutrition regimen, possibly at home. The results of surgical treatment (resection of the small intestine) of CIIP are disappointing.

Intermezzo 18

The ileocaecal sphincter

At the juncture between ileum and colon the circular muscle is thicker. Both circular and longitudinal muscle form a sphincter—the ileocaecal sphincter (or ileocaecal valve). This structure protrudes somewhat into the caecum and can easily be seen upon colonoscopic examination. Few researchers have studied the ileocaecal sphincter to date. The reason is that it is difficult to access for research purposes.

The ileocaecal sphincter is closed at rest and the resting pressure is so low in man that some researchers have not been able to find a high-pressure zone in it. It has been suggested that the most important function of the ileocaecal sphincter is to prevent colo-ileal reflux and bacterial overgrowth of the small intestine. In patients in whom, for one or another reason, the sphincter is removed (ileocaecal resection, mostly because of Crohn's disease), bacterial overgrowth of the last portion of the small intestine is indeed observed more often. After ileocaecal resection in dogs the terminal ileum in the fasting state produced more contractions than previously, whilst the long intervals of motor quiescence (phase I) of the MMC

were absent. Specific dysmotilities of the ileocaecal valve have not (yet) been described.

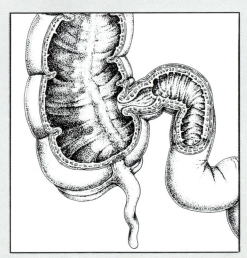

Figure 76: The ileocaecal sphincter.

Conclusion

In the past few years an increasing number of functional disorders of the small intestine have been identified. In some patients these are attended by disorders of the stomach or large intestine (gastroduodenal dysfunction, IBS). Some functional disorders of the small intestine are relatively mild but others are life-threatening (ileus, CIIP). Timely detection of these disorders can spare the patient considerable inconvenience. Treatment is often difficult, although new prokinetic drugs offer more possibilities than previously.

References

Camilleri M, Brown ML, Malagelada JR. Impaired transit of chyme in chronic intestinal pseudo-obstruction. Correction by cisapride. Gastroenterology 1986; 91: 619–626

Cann PA, Read NW, Brown C, e.a. Irritable bowel syndrome: relationship of disorder in the transit of a single solid meal to symptom patterns. Gut 1983; 24: 405–411

Kellow JE, Phillips SF. Altered small bowel motility in irritable bowel syndrome is correlated with symptoms. Gastroenterology 1987; 92: 1886–1893

Malagelada JR, Stanghellini V. Manometric evaluation of functional upper gut symptoms. Gastroenterology 1985; 88: 1223–1231

Malagelada JR, Camilleri M, Stanghellini V. Manometric diagnosis of gastrointestinal motility disorders. New York: Thieme, 1986

Read NW, Al-Jabani MN, Holgate AM, Barber DC, Edwards CA. Simultaneous measurement of gastric emptying, small bowel residence and colonic filling of a solid meal by the use of the gamma camera. Gut 1986; 27: 300–308

The large intestine

When the motility of the large intestine becomes disordered, for whatever reason, constipation, diarrhoea or pain can result. In this chapter we address motility disturbances of the large intestine, and focus on a troublesome disorder—the Irritable Bowel Syndrome (IBS).

Introduction

The most important functions of the large intestine are to resorb water and electrolytes from the liquid chyme that enters it from the small intestine and to store faecal material temporarily. The contractions of the colon have an important part to play in this respect. The faeces that are finally excreted consist largely of bacteria, which account for up to 50–60% of the faecal content.

When the movements of the large intestine become disordered, for whatever reason, constipation, diarrhoea, pain or a combination of these can result. When abdominal pain is present with (relatively mild) constipation, diarrhoea or alternating constipation and diarrhoea, and when no clear cause can be found, the condition is called Irritable Bowel Syndrome (IBS). IBS is the most frequent diagnosis made in connection with disorders of the large intestine. In many patients with IBS the contractions of the large intestine are more powerful than normal and some of these patients have spasms. But in some patients with IBS the contractions are insufficient in number and strength. These motility disorders can be caused by psychological factors or by food, but it is now thought that there is also a large group of IBS patients with a primary dysmotility. In addition to IBS other primary and secondary motility disorders can cause constipation, diarrhoea or abdominal pain (Figure 77).

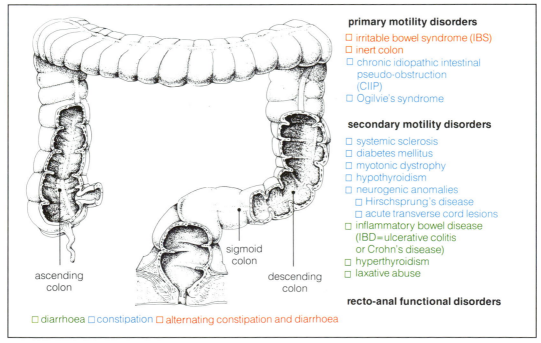

primary motility disorders

☐ irritable bowel syndrome (IBS)
☐ inert colon
☐ chronic idiopathic intestinal
  pseudo-obstruction
  (CIIP)
☐ Ogilvie's syndrome

secondary motility disorders

☐ systemic sclerosis
☐ diabetes mellitus
☐ myotonic dystrophy
☐ hypothyroidism
☐ neurogenic anomalies
  ☐ Hirschsprung's disease
  ☐ acute transverse cord lesions
☐ inflammatory bowel disease
  (IBD=ulcerative colitis
  or Crohn's disease)
☐ hyperthyroidism
☐ laxative abuse

recto-anal functional disorders

ascending colon

sigmoid colon

descending colon

☐ diarrhoea ☐ constipation ☐ alternating constipation and diarrhoea

Figure 77: Primary and secondary motor disorders of the large intestine.

Anatomy

The structure of the large intestine

The large intestine is about 1.5 m long in man. Generally it has more flexures in the abdominal cavity than is indicated by schematic diagrams. The longitudinal muscle of the stomach, small intestine and rectum pass over the entire circumference of these organs but the longitudinal muscle of the large intestine splits into three longitudinal bands called the taeniae. The circular muscle extends over the entire circumference.

---

stimulate motility:
— gastrin
— cholecystokinin
— substance P
— enkephalins

inhibit motility:
— glucagon
— vasoactive intestinal
  polypeptide (VIP)
— secretin

Table 6: Hormones (and neuropeptides) that affect the large intestine.

Innervation of the large intestine

As in the stomach and small intestine there is a dense network of nerve cells and nerve fibres in the wall of the large intestine, the myenteric plexus and the submucosa. These nerve cells act on one another and receive input from the extrinsic system, which consists of a sympathetic and a parasympathetic component. The parasympathetic fibres that regulate the right colon reach this part via the vagal nerve and the parasympathetic fibres that regulate the left colon reach it via the pelvic splanchnic nerves. The sympathetic fibres innervate the colon via the perivascular plexuses (Figure 10, p. 32). The motility of the large intestine is also controlled by a number of hormones (Table 6).

The movements of the large intestine

The smooth muscle cells

The movements of the large intestine are more complex (and less well understood) than those of the stomach or small intestine. Whereas there are regular, rhythmic depolarizations (the electrical control activity, ECA, p. 42) of the smooth muscle in the stomach and small intestine, there are uniquely irregular potential fluctuations in the large intestine (Figure 78). Also, the movements of the large intestine are more variable than those of the stomach and small intestine. In the stomach and small intestine peristaltic contractions spread distally along the entire length, but in the large intestine the contractions are fundamentally different.

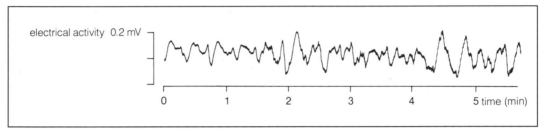

Figure 78: Electrical activity of the human colon, recorded with a mucosal electrode. Irregular activity, in the form of potential fluctuations, is evident.

Types of contractions

Two principal types of contractions can be identified in the large intestine: haustral contractions and mass contractions.

◆ Haustral contractions cause ring-like constrictions along the large intestine. The colon owes its characteristic exterior to this activity (Figure 79). The location of these constrictions varies continuously. The contractions are slow, most of them lasting a few dozen seconds. Intraluminal manometry reveals them to be pressure waves of variable duration and amplitude (Figure 86, p. 160). The most important function of the haustral contractions is to mix and grind the colonic contents, as a result of which these are extensively exposed to the mucosa. In this way the resorption of water and electrolytes is promoted.

◆ With mass contractions, the circular muscle contracts over a larger portion of the large intestine. In addition, the receiving portion of the intestine is often relaxed beforehand. The contractions travel distally at a speed of about 1 cm/s. As a result the colonic contents are pushed toward the anus. Mass contractions in the sigmoid lead to defaecation, but this response is not always provoked. The defaecation urge can of course be suppressed. Mass contractions occur only a few times per day. They are therefore rarely disclosed by a radiographic examination (Figure 80). On the other hand, they can be readily observed by means of 24-hour manometric recording (Figure 81).

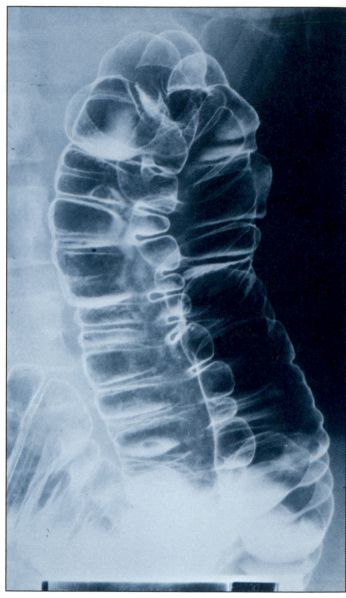

Figure 79: Radiograph of a part of the colon, enhanced by double contrast (air and barium). The segmental, haustral contractions are clearly defined and give the colon its characteristic exterior.

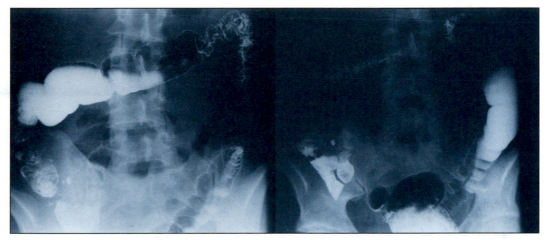

Figure 80: Mass movement in the colon, recorded on a radiograph with contrast medium.

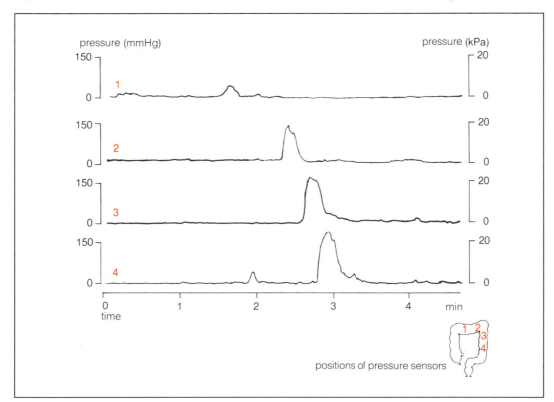

Figure 81: Mass movement in the colon, recorded by means of intraluminal manometry.
A large pressure wave travelling distally is well defined.

Postprandial and interdigestive activity

When there is food in the stomach (i.e. in the postprandial state), the motility patterns of stomach and small and large intestines are different from when the food is eliminated from the stomach (i.e. in the interdigestive phase).

◆ A few minutes **after the meal** the electrical and the motor activity rise sharply (Figure 87, p. 162). This activity lasts 30–60 minutes and constitutes the gastrocolic response (or reflex). During this response the colon produces additional haustral contractions and sometimes mass contractions. These mass contractions can provoke a (sometimes embarrassing) defaecation urge after the meal. At the very start of the meal additional gastrin and cholecystokinin are released and it is suggested that these hormones elicit the gastrocolic response. This response must not be confused with the postprandial pattern of the stomach and small intestine. It rarely lasts longer than 1 hour, whilst the postprandial pattern, depending on the quantity and kind of food in the meal, can last longer than 5 hours.

◆ In the **fasting state** the MMC is active in the stomach and small intestine (p. 46). In the large intestine there is no equivalent of the MMC. If the MMC also occurred in the large intestine, this would be cleaned out every 1.5 hours in the fasting state (e.g. at night) and defaecation would occur*. For the resorption of water and electrolytes, however, it is important that the faecal material should remain in the large intestine (generally from 1 to 3 days). In a normal feeding pattern, therefore, the large intestine is never empty (Figure 82).

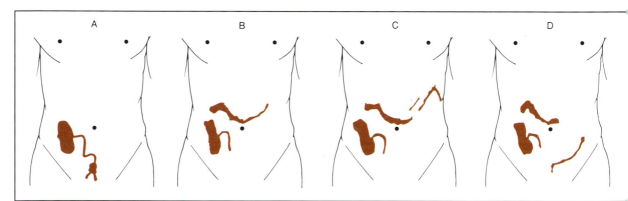

Figure 82: The transport of material down the large intestine and the effect of the following meal. A: 5 hours after a "barium meal" (barium indicated by brown). Immediately after A, another meal was consumed. B: 10 minutes after this second meal. C: 15 minutes after second meal. D: 17 minutes after second meal. (Reproduced with permission, from Ritchie, 1968.)

* Night-time diarrhoea of this type occurs in the early months after a (sub)total colectomy (with an ileorectal or ileoanal anastomosis).

Intermezzo 19
Examination of the large intestine

◆ Radiographic examination of the large intestine (with a barium enema) is important not only for the exclusion of organic abnormalities but also for the analysis of the movements of the large intestine. **Spasms** or **dilation** of the large intestine can often be clearly observed by means of a radiographic examination. If dilation has occurred there is often atony of the smooth muscle. Giving the patient pellets or rings to swallow and following these on radiographs permits the measurement of **transit time** (Figure 126, p. 285). If these particles reside in the large intestine too long, the diagnosis of constipation can be objectively confirmed and in addition it can be seen where the beads are held up in the colon. By means of cineradiography (defaecography) the **defaecation process** can be observed (Chapter 11).

◆ **Endoscopy** of the large intestine (colonoscopy) is often an appropriate means of demonstrating organic abnormalities. By means of this technique it is also possible to observe spasms clearly.

◆ **Scintigraphy** is a method suitable for the measurement of transport through the large intestine. Radioactive material is introduced into the right colon by means of a catheter or special coated tablets and it is then followed. However, this technique has so far been limited to research activities.

◆ **Manometry** is used to register the movements of the large intestine. However, it is not yet possible to make a firm diagnosis by means of this technique; considerable variation in colonic movements is also found in healthy controls. In principle, prolonged (24-hour) manometry appears to be suitable for detecting occasionally occurring motility disorders. However, manometry of the large intestine is still a research tool.

The symptoms of dysmotility of the large intestine

In taking the history of a patient with colon symptoms one should ask for details of the symptoms pain, constipation and diarrhoea. If constipation and diarrhoea are present, one should focus on consistency, quantity and composition of the faeces. This information provides important indications for the diagnosis.

Pain
The pain from motility disorders can result from strong contractions (spasms)

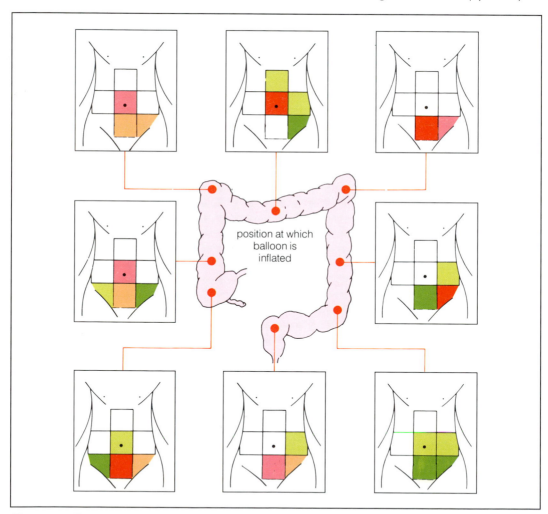

Figure 83: Relationship between the location at which the pain is felt in the abdomen and the site at which a balloon is inflated in the colon. (Reproduced with permission, from Swarbrick et al., 1980.)

or stretching of the intestine due to the accumulation of faeces and gas. Burning, chronic pain or pain on being touched points to hypomotility, in which case the intestinal wall is stretched by faeces or gas. Crampy, intermittent pain, on the other hand, tends to be indicative of spasms or hypermotility. The patient can feel the pain at different points in his or her abdomen, and sometimes in the back, chest or thighs. The location of the pain does not always correspond to the location in the colon of the abnormality (Figure 83). It is typical of colonic pain that it often subsides after a productive defaecation. If the patient feels the pain uniquely in the upper abdomen, the cause should generally be sought in the stomach, although in a number of patients it lies in the large intestine. Pain in the upper abdomen is of course not a rare occurrence in patients with constipation. Even if the pain intensifies shortly after the meal, it may arise from the colon, due to the gastrocolic response.

Constipation
The diagnostic criteria for constipation are as follows: a low defaecation frequency, a low faeces production, hard faeces, a feeling of incomplete intestinal emptying and the necessity of overstraining in order to defaecate. Even for a symptom as frequent as constipation there is no generally accepted set of criteria. However, a defaecation frequency of less than once every two days and an average faecal weight of less than 100 grams are adopted as a rule of thumb.

Diarrhoea
The definition of diarrhoea poses similar problems. When a patient complains of diarrhoea it is not always clear what he or she means by this term. For example, some patients with diarrhoea produce small quantities of relatively normal faeces several times a day and others a larger quantity of loose stool. In general no clear relationship has been established between defaecation frequency and faecal consistency.

Diagnostic examination

For the examination of patients with abdominal pain, constipation or diarrhoea there are no general guidelines. It is particularly important with these patients, however, that the examination should focus on the situation of the individual patient. For example, if a 60-year-old patient complains of constipation that has been present for a few months, colonic carcinoma is a more plausible diagnosis than for a 25-year-old patient who has had intermittent abdominal symptoms for many years. On the basis of the history and a physical examination, the nonsuspected and suspected causes can be preliminarily sorted out (cf. pp. 221–223). A simple laboratory analysis (BSE, Hb, occult blood in the stool) can facilitate the diagnosis. Accumulation of faecal matter can be seen by means of a plain film of the abdomen without administration of a contrast medium, with the patient supine. Colonoscopy or a radiographic examination may be appropriate if there is doubt about the existence of organic disturbances. Because diarrhoea can result from many different disorders, examination by a specialist is often recommended for patients in whom this symptom is severe. Only after elimination of other possible causes of the symptoms can supplementary motility studies be considered. The determination of colonic transit time is often the first investigation to consider.

The disorders

Constipation, diarrhoea or abdominal pain can be caused by a number of organic anomalies (Table 7). Disordered colonic motor activity can arise secondarily to a number of disorders, such as diabetes mellitus, systemic sclerosis, hypo- or hyperthyroidism, ulcerative colitis and Crohn's disease. Excessive use of laxatives can also lead to chronic diarrhoea. Only after elimination of these factors as causes, can it be concluded that the patient may have a primary motility disorder. Constipation and diarrhoea can also be caused by a rectoanal disorder (e.g. see anismus in Chapter 11).

IBS
The most frequently diagnosed primary motility disorder of the colon is IBS. This syndrome is defined as a disorder that manifests itself by abdominal pain, constipation and diarrhoea (Figure 81) or alternating constipation and diarrhoea (Figure 81) and that cannot be causally explained by other disorders. However, it is impossible to exclude all disorders as being causal because the procedure involved would be too stressful for the patient and take too much time. In practice the diagnosis of IBS is made after elimination of a limited number of obvious disorders (cf. Figure 77 and Table 7); genuine diagnostic criteria for the IBS have not been established.

IBS: constipation and motor activity
In IBS patients with constipation an excess of colonic haustral contractions (hyperhaustration) is often observed,

	constipation	diarrhoea	abdominal pain
— IBD (Crohn's disease and ulcerative colitis)		+ +	+
— diverticular disease	+		+ +
— colon carcinoma	+ +		+
— intestinal infections		+ +	+
— peptic ulcer			+ +
— cholelithiasis			+ +
— lactose intolerance		+ +	+
— food intolerance and food allergy		+ +	+
— pancreatic cancer		+	+ +
— coeliac disease		+ +	

Table 7: Differential diagnosis: the most prevalent disorders that are accompanied by constipation, diarrhoea or abdominal pain and that must be differentiated from IBS.

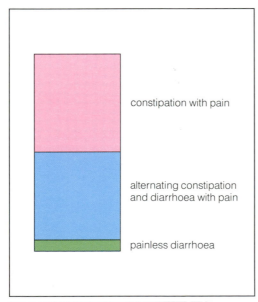

Figure 84: Relative frequency of symptoms of IBS in patients that are referred to a gastroenterologist.

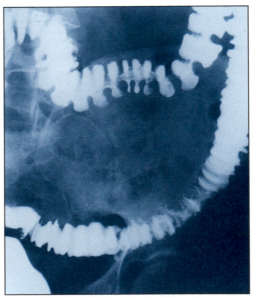

Figure 85: Typical spasms and hyperhaustration of the sigmoid colon in a patient with IBS, as recorded by means of a radiographic examination.

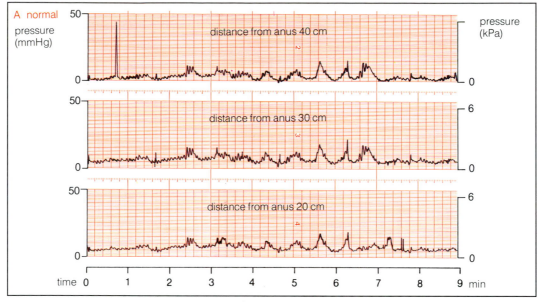

Figure 86A: Manometric recordings of the sigmoid colon in a healthy volunteer. The pressure waves are simultaneous. No compartments are formed in the lumen in which pressure can build up.

which gives rise to a narrowing of the sigmoid colon.

This can be seen by means of a radiographic, endoscopic or manometric examination (Figures 85 and 86A). In the stomach and small intestine the movements are primarily propulsive. In hypermotility therefore the food is transported more rapidly through the stomach and intestine. In the large intestine, however, the movements are primarily haustral waves and non-propulsive. Hypermotility in the large intestine can therefore lead to constipation. In the narrowest segment of the large intestine, the sigmoid colon, in particular, extra contractions hold up faecal transport rather than promote it. Patients with IBS sometimes have an abnormal postprandial response; the gastrocolic response occurs in them later but persists longer (Figure 87). This observation possibly explains the symptom of pain after meals in some patients. Neither in IBS nor in other motility disorders have unequivocal abnormalities of the electrical control activity (ECA) been found.

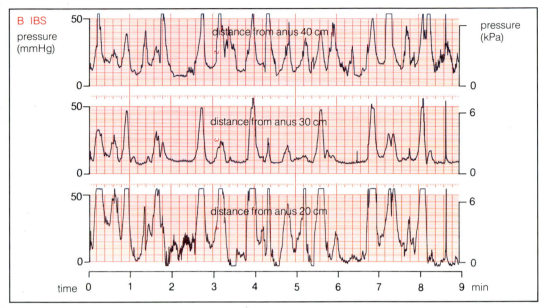

Figure 86B: Manometric recordings of the sigmoid colon in a patient with IBS. There is an increase in the amplitude of the pressure waves. In the patient the pressure waves are not simultaneous (cf. Figure 86A).

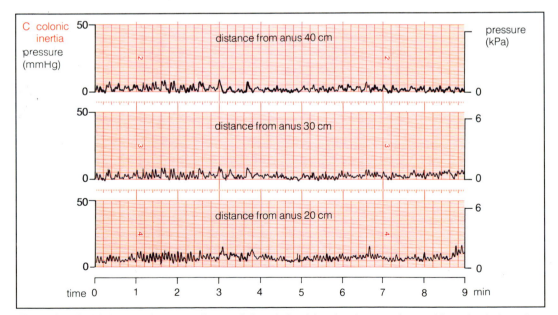

Figure 86C: Manometric recordings of the sigmoid colon in a patient with colonic inertia.

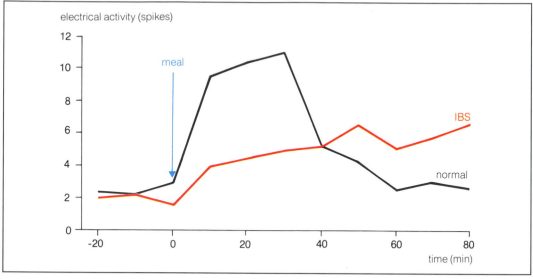

Figure 87: The gastrocolic response in healthy volunteers and patients with IBS. In these patients this response starts later and lasts longer. (Reproduced with permission, from Sullivan et al. 1978.)

IBS: diarrhoea and motor activity

Patients with IBS sometimes excrete a small quantity of slightly pasty stool several times a day. The total quantity of stool is not or hardly increased. These patients can generally sleep through the night. This pattern contrasts with that of patients with diarrhoea caused by infections of the large intestine. These patients have more stool per day than is normal and are often awoken at night by the defaecation urge. In IBS patients in whom diarrhoea is the dominant symptom, decreased motility of the sigmoid colon is often observed. However, this finding cannot be used as a diagnostic criterion since there is a large overlap with controls. The diarrhoea is probably provoked by a hypersensitivity of the rectum; small quantities of faeces in the rectum are enough to elicit the defaecation urge (see Chapter 11).

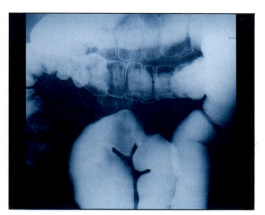

Figure 88: Radiograph of the large intestine in colonic inertia.

Intermezzo 20
Defining the term IBS

About half the patients referred to a gastroenterologist suffer from IBS. It is sometimes tacitly assumed that this diagnosis refers to a homogeneous group of patients. It is much more likely, however, that IBS comprises a number of disorders for which we do not yet know the causes. The IBS is therefore a mixed bag of disorders. Some even propose to abandon the term IBS altogether and speak of "non-organically explained abdominal complaints". How one names the syndrome is a relatively trivial matter. What is important however is that the following conditions be fulfilled:

◆ severe or treatable disorders should always be excluded;
◆ the disorder must be described to the patient in the appropriate terms; in this way he or she will have some idea of the disorder and will not become unduly anxious;
◆ the term used for the disorder must be correctly interpreted by medical colleagues.

Perhaps IBS is provisionally not such a bad umbrella term for the abnormalities that it covers. It is to be expected that in the future abnormalities will be identified that will no longer be attributed to the IBS, and a smaller and smaller group of patients will still be considered to suffer from "the IBS".

Disorders marked by severe constipation

Some patients have very severe constipation because their colon produces too few contractions. This condition is referred to as colonic inertia ("slow colon"). Radiographic examination of the colon, discloses that it is wide and usually also long with few haustra (Figure 88). Manometry reveals that there are hardly any significant contractions (Figure 86C). The cause of inert colon is not known. However, it has been established that the number of neurons in the intramural plexus of the colon is diminished. It is still unclear whether the small number of neurons is the cause or the result of the prolonged constipation. Also **chronic idiopathic intestinal pseudo-obstruction** (CIIP) can also be accompanied by a decrease in the number of contractions of the large intestine. This picture is similar to that of colonic inertia. An uncommon form of severe colonic atony with acute onset is **Ogilvie's syndrome**. The origin of this disorder is not known.

Treatment of primary motility disorders

IBS patients are particularly in need of an explanation of their disorder and reassurance; if the patient is reassured, he or she can better tolerate the symptoms and sometimes they disappear. It cannot be concluded, however, that the symptoms are "therefore" psychogenic. On the other hand, stress, for example, can transiently exacerbate the symptoms, probably via the autonomic nervous system.

Constipation: fibre, laxatives, spasmolytics or prokinetics?

A treatment is chosen on the basis of the nature and severity of the symptoms, the effect of previous treatments and the information provided by radiographic examination (and, when appropriate, manometry).

◆ Constipation is often reduced by a **fibre-rich diet**. Fibres enlarge the volume of the faecal matter and retain water. In addition, bacteria digest fibre, thereby increasing the volume of the bacteria in the faeces. Sometimes bulking agents, like psysillium seed or sterculia gum, are beneficial.

◆ If there is evidence of hypermotility (spasms) of the large intestine, **spasmolytics** are often used. For IBS, generally the relaxants mebeverine or pinaverium are used. These substances act directly on the smooth muscle.

◆ If there is evidence of hypomotility of the large intestine (inertia) and if the effect of fibre is not sufficient, other **laxatives** may be desirable. The water content of the faecal matter can be increased and the faeces can be made softer by means of osmotically active laxatives like magnesium compounds (magnesium oxide, magnesium sulphate or magnesium citrate) and lactulose. In addition there are contact laxatives, which stimulate the mucosa of the large intestine, thereby increasing the number of contractions it makes. To this class belong bisacodyl and enemas.

◆ If there is evidence of hypomotility it can be attempted to stimulate the motility of the large intestine with prokinetics. It would then be inherently logical to use prokinetics (e.g. cisapride) that release acetylcholine, but the effect of this substance has not yet been fully investigated.

◆ Exceptionally constipation can be so severe that **surgery** is appropriate. This can happen with colonic inertia, CIIP and Ogilvie's syndrome. The surgical options are partial, subtotal or total colectomy. Surgery is never performed for IBS.

Diarrhoea

Supplementary fibre is generally not a desirable treatment for diarrhoea. Instead, IBS patients with diarrhoea are treated with bulking agents. Because these substances bind water, they improve faecal consistency. The diarrhoea itself can be reduced by loperamide.

Intermezzo 21
Secondary motility disorders of the large intestine

Secondary constipation or diarrhoea develops in some other disorders (Figure 77). We shall mention the most important of these.

◆ In diabetes mellitus constipation is observed fairly frequently as an accompanying complaint. Patients with **diabetes mellitus** do not have a gastrocolic response. Drugs like cisapride and metoclopramide, which stimulate intestinal contractions by releasing acetylcholine, stimulate colon activity in these patients. This indicates that a neuronal disorder in diabetes mellitus (neuropathy) is a cause of dysmotility.

◆ Patients with **systemic sclerosis** do not have the postprandial response. Unlike diabetics, however, systemic sclerosis patients sometimes do not react to prokinetics that release acetylcholine. It is probable that in an early phase of the disease mainly neurological deficits are present and that later the smooth muscles are dysfunctional.

◆ **Ulcerative colitis and Crohn's disease** are forms of Inflammatory Bowel Disease (IBD). The term IBD is often used because ulcerative colitis and Crohn's disease often cannot be differentiated from one another. In IBD the motor activity of the large intestine can become secondarily disordered. During an exacerbation of the inflammation the contractions of the affected colonic regions are considerably diminished. In these patients the gastrocolic response is also diminished. After remission of the inflammation a normal motor activity can be re-established.

◆ The contractions of the large intestine and the defaecation pattern can also become severely disordered after **nerve lesions**. After an acute transverse cord lesion the most important problem is that the patient can no longer voluntarily contract and relax the circular muscle of the anus and the abdominal muscles. As a result he or she can no longer strain nor retain faeces. After a vagotomy parasympathetic control of the right colon is lost. After a truncal vagotomy diarrhoea often occurs. In principle this development can be explained by the effects of vagotomy on the stomach and small intestine; whether the absence of parasympathetic innervation of the large intestine also plays a part is unclear. In interventions of the minor pelvis, such as extirpation of the uterus, the pelvic splanchnic nerves are sometimes severed accidentally, which brings about atony of the left colon and constipation.

Conclusion

We are gradually gaining more insight into motility disorders of the large intestine. Both too many contractions (spasms) and too few contractions (atony) of the large intestine can bring about constipation. It is likely that this also applies to diarrhoea. In most cases of abdominal pain with mild constipation, the diagnosis is IBS. In general a patient with IBS is given dietary advice. If this proves ineffective, a rational strategy involving the use of bulking agents, laxatives, spasmolytics, prokinetics or antidiarrhoeal agents should be worked out on the basis of the symptoms and the results of supplementary examinations. Some patients suffer from severe forms of constipation (e.g. colonic inertia, CIIP or Olgilvie's syndrome). In addition, motility disturbances of the large intestine can arise secondarily to other disorders.

In the past 10 years more has been learned about the normal movements of the large intestine. And yet many questions remain unanswered. We should like to know for example precisely how the haustral and mass contractions come about. How does the faecal matter affect the contractions of the large intestine? And what is the exact role of the parasympathetic nervous system? If we knew the answers to these questions, a better targeted approach to dysmotility of the large intestine would be possible. Notwithstanding, however, the new investigation methods permit a more precise characterization of patients with colon symptoms. It can now be investigated in this group whether given motility patterns of the large intestine are disordered. By means of 24-hour manometry occasional irregularities can be detected. Use of the new techniques for investigation will substantially improve the diagnosis and treatment of patients with constipation, diarrhoea or abdominal pain.

References

Christensen J. Motility of the colon. In: Johnson LR, ed. Physiology of the gastrointestinal tract. New York: Raven Press, 1987: 665–693

Manning AP, e.a. Towards a positive diagnosis of the irritable bowel. Br Med J 1978; 2: 633–636

Narducci F, e.a. Twenty-four hour manometric recording of colonic motor activity in healthy man. Gut 1978; 28: 17–25

Ritchie JA. Colonic motor activity and bowel function. Gut 1968; 9: 442–456

Ritchie JA. Pain in IBS. Pract Gastroenterol 1979; 3: 16–21

Smith B. Pathologic changes in the colon produced by anthraquinone purgatives. Dis Colon Rectum 1973; 13: 455–463

Sullivan MA, e.a. Colonic myoelectric activity in irritable bowel syndrome. Effect of eating and anti-cholinergics. N Engl J Med 1978; 298: 878–883

Swarbrick ET, e.a. Site of pain from the irritable bowel. Lancet 1980; 2: 443–447

FROM OESOPHAGUS TO ANUS

Rectum, anus and pelvic floor

Traditionally constipation and incontinence have been considered to be "troublesome" disorders that are difficult to treat. And yet there must be a causal factor such that some patients cannot expel faeces and others cannot retain them. Almost invariably this factor has to do with an anomaly of the anatomy, innervation or motility of the colon, rectum, anus and pelvic floor. The art consists in identifying this pathology. In addition there is a group of patients with severe (often difficult to understand) perianal or anorectal pain.

Introduction

The anorectal region and the pelvic floor are anatomically fairly complex structures, consisting of smooth and striated muscle. The actions of these muscles must be highly co-ordinated in order to retain and expel the faeces voluntarily. The ability to perceive that the rectum is full, to retain the rectal contents and to choose a suitable moment for defaecation is called faecal (anal) continence.

Because retaining the faeces and postponing defaecation require good co-ordination between many muscles, the weakest step in the process determines the final action. Both the anorectum and the pelvic floor are liable to dysfunction, so that the umbrella term "pelvic floor syndromes" has been adopted. Another disorder of the anorectum or pelvic floor is the frequently severe anorectal pain.

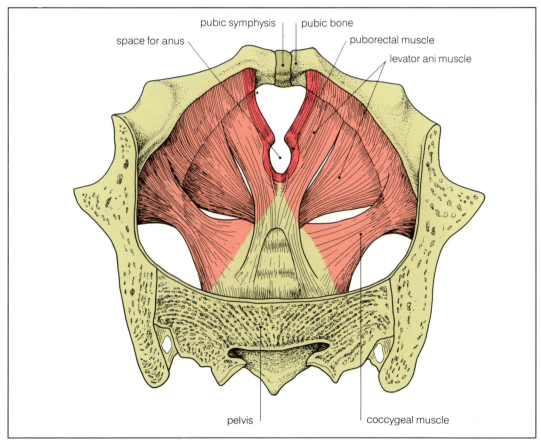

Figure 89: The position of the muscles of the pelvic floor.

Anatomy

The rectum

The rectum is the continuation of the large intestine. The longitudinal muscle of the colon (and therefore of the sigmoid colon too) extends in three strips (taeniae). But at the end of the sigmoid colon these strips fan out to form the continuous longitudinal muscle layer of the rectum. The rectum is 10–15 cm long and passes inferiorly from the rectosigmoid junction at the third sacral vertebra to the anal canal. The rectum lies at the back of the abdominal cavity, against the sacral vertebrae, except for the most distal part, (cf. Figure 91).

The anal canal

The most distal part of the rectum narrows at the juncture of rectum and anus, which is also called the anorectal ring (Figure 90). The anorectal ring is

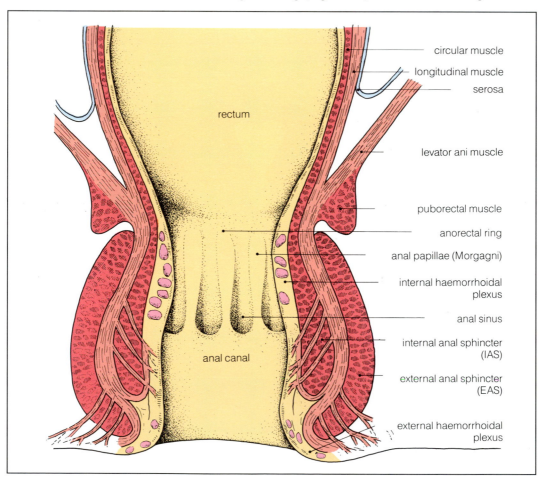

Figure 90: Detail of the structure of the anal region.

Intermezzo 22
Study methods

◆ **Manometry** is an important technique for studying the activity of the rectum and anus. Manometry permits different types of measurements:
— the anal pressure profile (Figure 94)
— the rectoanal inhibition reflex (p. 182, Figure 95)
— the rectal compliance (Intermezzo 23); while this measurement is performed the rectal sensitivity can also be determined
— the maximum squeeze pressure (especially of the EAS).
By means of manometry prolonged recordings can be made of the contractions of the sigmoid colon, rectum and anal canal, even in outpatients. It is possible to measure the pressure at several positions simultaneously.

◆ The **expulsion test** is suitable for directly investigating whether a patient is able to expel faeces. For this purpose water-filled balloons or soft silicone boluses of different diameters and shapes are used. These are inserted into the rectum of the patient, who is asked to try to expel them.

◆ The **saline infusion test**. This method is used for determining whether the person can retain water in the rectum, and if so, how much. By means of a small catheter, physiological saline (37°C) is pumped slowly into the patient's rectum. The patient is instructed to retain as much as possible. The time at which the solution begins to leak and the quantity are noted.

◆ **Sensitivity measurement**. The sensitivity of the mucosa of the rectum and anus can also be determined by electrical stimulation of the mucosa by electrodes.

◆ **Defaecography**. With this method the defaecation process can be followed as it occurs naturally (p.284).

◆ By means of **electromyography** the pattern of contraction of individual muscle groups can be recorded. The activity of the EAS can be globally measured by placement of electrodes on the skin and detailed measurements can be performed by insertion of (needle) electrodes. For the EMG of the IAS and the muscles of the pelvic floor needle-electrodes are needed; for the IAS very thin electrodes (diameter: 0.025 mm) are used.

formed by the proximal border of the internal anal sphincter (IAS) and external anal sphincter (EAS). The puborectal muscle is also located here. The anal canal itself is 3–4 cm long.

◆ The **IAS** is a distal continuation of the circular smooth muscle of the rectum. In the anus there is a thicker layer of smooth circular muscle than in the rectum. The IAS is almost always contracted, relaxing in response to certain stimulations only and then for only a short interval.

◆ The **longitudinal smooth muscle** of the rectum passes along the wall of the anal canal. The striated longitudinal muscle of the puborectal muscle extends through the same region (Figure 90). The longitudinal muscle is therefore partly smooth and partly striated. It passes like a septum between the IAS and the EAS. The fibres of this muscle are attached to elastic fibres that fan out into a number of separate strips that pass through the EAS or the IAS and attach to the skin.

◆ The **EAS**, a striated muscle, lies more distally, partially surrounding the IAS. Ordinarily the EAS has a resting tone, which the person increases by squeezing and lowers by defaecating (or straining without defaecating).

◆ The **haemorrhoidal plexus** also lies in the anal canal (Figure 90). It consists of folds with venous structures that function as cavernous bodies. They contribute to the water- and air-tightness of the anal canal.

The pelvic floor
The pelvic floor is built up out of a number of muscles (Figure 89). We shall mention here the muscles that play an important part in continence and defaecation. The **levator ani muscle** is the large muscle of the ventral part of the pelvic floor. An important constituent of this muscle is the **puborectal muscle**, which passes around the rectum in U-shaped fashion. Most of the time the levator ani and the puborectal muscle have a resting tone. The latter muscle therefore pulls the rectum forward and reduces the anorectal angle (Figure 91). Owing to its resting tone the levator ani maintains the pelvic floor and the anus in an upward position. During defaecation the levator ani and the puborectal muscle relax. The **coccygeal muscle** is the large muscle of the dorsal part of the pelvic floor. Together with the IAS, the EAS keeps the anal canal closed. This sphincter is situated under (distally from) the puborectal muscle.

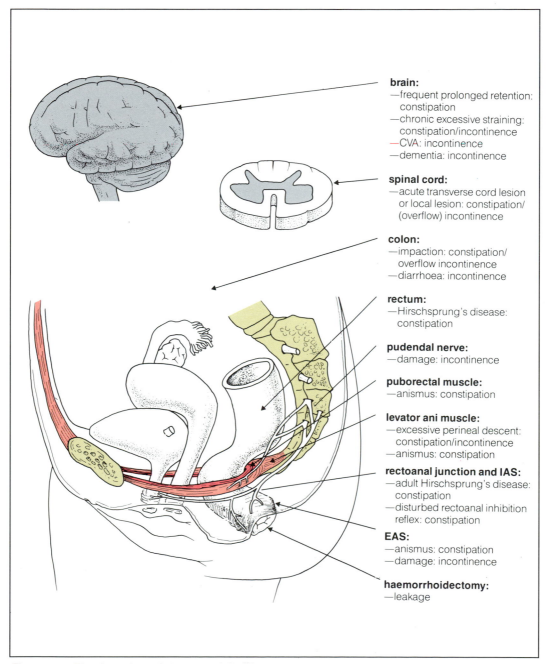

brain:
—frequent prolonged retention: constipation
—chronic excessive straining: constipation/incontinence
—CVA: incontinence
—dementia: incontinence

spinal cord:
—acute transverse cord lesion or local lesion: constipation/ (overflow) incontinence

colon:
—impaction: constipation/ overflow incontinence
—diarrhoea: incontinence

rectum:
—Hirschsprung's disease: constipation

pudendal nerve:
—damage: incontinence

puborectal muscle:
—anismus: constipation

levator ani muscle:
—excessive perineal descent: constipation/incontinence
—anismus: constipation

rectoanal junction and IAS:
—adult Hirschsprung's disease: constipation
—disturbed rectoanal inhibition reflex: constipation

EAS:
—anismus: constipation
—damage: incontinence

haemorrhoidectomy:
—leakage

Figure 91: The location of the most important organs of the lower abdomen. The sites at which disorders can provoke constipation and/or incontinence are also indicated.

Innervation

The innervation of the anus is complex and different from the innervation of the rest of the digestive tract (Figure 92). In the rectum there is a well-defined enteric nervous system with a myenteric and a submucosal plexus. But from the anectoral ring the density of the ganglion cells decreases distally. Below the dentate line they are absent. The **IAS** is controlled by the extrinsic autonomic nervous system (sympathetic and parasympathetic). The fibres of the nerves of this system also innervate the enteric nervous system (ENS), which in turn innervates the IAS. The sympathetic fibres arise from the lumbar level of the spinal cord (L5) and the postganglionic fibres reach the IAS via the hypogastric plexus and the pelvic plexus. The parasympathetic fibres arise from the sacral level of the spinal cord (S2-S4). They reach the rectum and anus via the pelvic plexus. Parasympathetic (cholinergic) fibres cause the IAS to relax, whereas sympathetic (noradrenergic) fibres cause it to contract through stimulation of α-receptors and cause it to relax by means of β-receptors. In addition, the IAS is intrinsically innervated from the myenteric plexus of the rectum and the proximal anal canal. The transmitters of the ENS that relax the IAS are likely to be adenosine triphosphate (ATP) and vasoactive intestinal polypeptide (VIP). The **EAS** is innervated via the pudendal nerve, which leaves from the sacral level of the spinal cord. The **other muscles** of the pelvis are innervated by the pudendal nerve. The **sensory cells** are located in the wall of the rectum. These react to distension of the rectal wall.

Sensory cells in the proximal canal also react to the composition of the rectal contents. These sensors affect the ENS, but their information also reaches the brain. The conducting fibres pass amongst the parasympathetic splanchnic fibres. Via these fibres one feels a defaecation urge and perceives whether there are faeces or gas above the anal canal. The muscles of the pelvic floor also contain sensory cells. These can play a role in the perception of rectal filling.

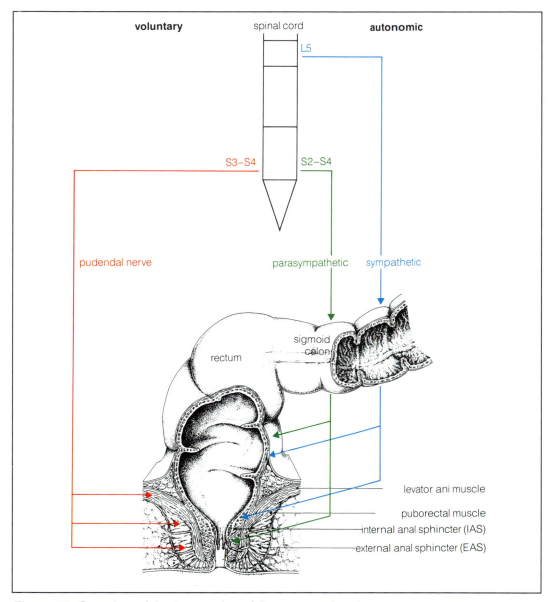

Figure 92: Overview of the innervation of the anorectal region.

The normal movements of rectum, anus and pelvic floor

Movements of the rectum: Delivery from the colon

Ordinarily the rectum is empty most of the time. From time to time only, faeces or gas from the colon arrive in the rectum. When the rectum is full, it is perceived that (1) something is present, (2) a certain quantity is present (a slight or intense urge) and (3) a certain material is present (faeces or gas). It is possible that this perception occurs only after the rectal contents have reached the anorectal juncture (see below). One then consciously decides whether or not to defaecate. If one decides not to defaecate, the material (faeces or gas) is transported back to the sigmoid colon.

Tonic contractions of the rectum

In the rectum there are tonic and phasic contractions. Ordinarily the rectum is almost empty. In this state a low tonic intraluminal resting pressure is present (about 0.8 kPa [6 mmHg]). When the rectum is full, the pressure increases somewhat (Figure 93). It is not yet clear whether this pressure comes about mainly as a result of elastic properties of the rectal wall or whether there are reflexes that control rectal pressure.

Phasic contractions of the rectum

Little research has as yet been done on the phasic contractions of the rectum but these appear to be complex. In only one publication have the results been presented of prolonged (19 hours) rectal monitoring in ambulatory volunteers.

Intermezzo 23
The compliance of the rectum

In order to study the activity of the rectum in patients it is sometimes useful to follow the pressure course in the rectum by progressive filling. Insertion of a catheter to whose tip a balloon has been tethered, permits measurement of this parameter. The intrarectal pressure is then manometrically recorded. The balloon is blown up (with air or water [37°C]) and the pressure measured (Figure 93A). After the pressure has been recorded, the balloon is allowed to empty, after an interval the balloon is filled with another volume (gradations about 10 ml). The change in pressure in the balloon when it is blown up outside the patient must of course also be determined. The difference between the pressure in the balloon outside the patient and the pressure in the balloon in the rectum is an indicator of the pressure built up in the rectum (Figure 93B). The ratio between volume and pressure is known as the compliance. Abnormalities can be detected by means of this method. Some persons have an inelastic rectum due, for example, to fibrosis induced by radiotherapy. An inelastic rectum has a deficient compliance. In contrast, a megarectum is too relaxed—its compliance is excessive. In healthy volunteers the compliance is generally between 30 and 80 ml/kPa (4–9 ml/mmHg or 3–7 ml/cm H_2O).

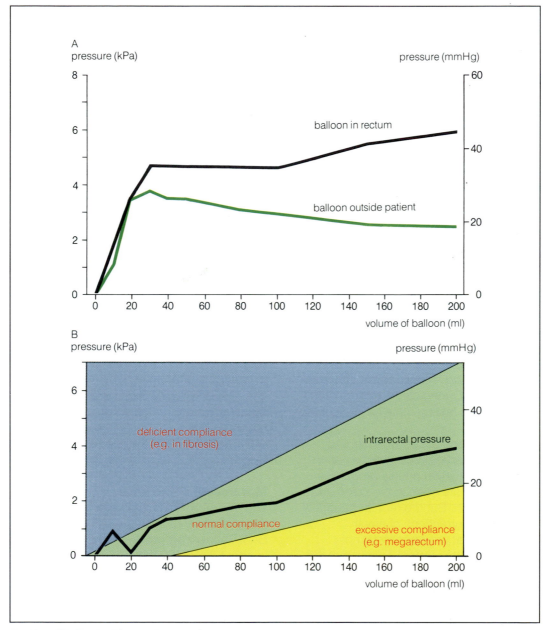

Figure 93: Compliance of the rectum. A: Pressure in the balloon when it is in the patient's rectum and outside the patient. B: Differential curve derived from the curves in A. This curve gives the compliance of the rectum. Normal values fall within the green zone, abnormal ones outside it.

The study described the following types of phasic contractions.

- ◆ Isolated prolonged contractions. During 10–20 sec the pressure rises slightly (to about 2 kPa = 15 mmHg). These contractions occur mainly in subjects in the waking state.

- ◆ Cluster contractions. Muscles in the rectum contract periodically (5–6 times per minute) during 1–2 minutes. This pattern occurs every 20–30 minutes. It is mainly observed after a meal.

- ◆ Powerful phasic contractions. About every 90 minutes another pattern of contractions occurs. (These contractions have the same period as the MMC.) About twice every minute the rectum produces a powerful contraction lasting 3–10 seconds. This activity is known as the rectal motor complex. During sleep these contractions are more regular and follow one another more rapidly. (During sleep most persons are in the fasting state for most of the time.)

It has long been asked whether and how the rectum participates in defaecation. During defaecation mainly propulsive contractions are seen in the colon and sigmoid colon. But the rectum generally produces contractions of small amplitude that are apparently not propagated. It therefore seems that the rectum is a passive relay canal. Also, if a balloon is blown up in the rectum, short-lasting contractions are observed. Finally, acute stress can bring about contractions of the smooth muscle of the rectal wall.

Sensors in the rectum and the anorectal zone

The sensors in the rectum and the anorectal junction seem quite different. In the rectum there are mainly stretch sensors, which detect whether filling has occurred. In the anorectal junction other sensors are found, which identify the composition of the rectal contents. Many rectal reflexes and contractions occur that escape our awareness. It is therefore assumed that some sensory information from the rectum is not accessible for conscious processing. At a certain moment, however, there is awareness that faeces or gas is present above the anal canal. Many persons can in addition feel whether the faecal matter is liquid or more solid. It is thought that the detection of filling and of the nature of the material is a component of the recto-anal inhibition reflex (see below). The sensory cells in the rectum react mainly to changes; after some time they adapt to a new pressure. If you resist a defaecation urge, after a while you will no longer feel it. It is likely that adaptation of the sensory cells plays a role in this respect.

Movements of the anus

The pressure that is registered in the anal canal is generated by the IAS and the EAS. The resting pressure of this canal is about 8 kPa (60 mmHg). (Figure 94). Of this about 7 kPa is contributed by the IAS and only 1 kPa by the EAS. The smooth muscle of the IAS can contract continuously without fatiguing but the striated EAS fatigues after about 1 minute of sustained contraction. Only the (voluntary) EAS is involved in anal squeezing. If this sphincter contracts more powerfully, the pressure in the anal canal can increase by a factor of about two.

Movement patterns of the IAS

In the resting state the smooth muscle of the (involuntary) IAS has an electrical control activity; the potential fluctuates with a frequency ranging from 6 to 20 cycles per minute. There is a frequency gradient in these oscillations. The highest frequency occurs distally. These oscillations increase in amplitude (but not in frequency) when the sphincter contracts. These fluctuations determine the contractions of the IAS and therefore the pressure in the anal canal. In the resting state the IAS is contracted. Phasic contractions are superimposed on the resting pressure.

◆ The resting pressure is characterized by small oscillations having an amplitude of about 1 kPa (7 mmHg). These oscillations are accompanied by fluctuations of the potential of the smooth muscle cells that range in frequency from 6 to 20 cycles per minute. Since the frequency is higher distally than proximally, any material that happens to be in the anal canal is pushed back into the rectum. This activity constitutes an additional mechanism for keeping the anal canal empty and preventing leakage.

◆ In addition, 40% of the time larger "ultra-slow waves" are observed. For about 30 seconds the pressure increases by 3–10 kPa (20–70 mmHg).

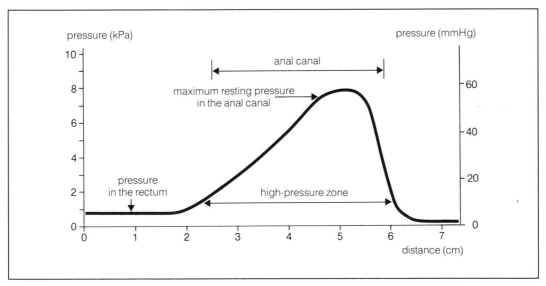

Figure 94: The rectum is characterized by a low pressure but at the level of the anal muscles the pressure is much higher. The above curve is obtained when a pressure sensor is inserted into the rectum and slowly pulled out. By means of this type of recording, the length of the (physiological) anal canal can be determined.

The (involuntary) IAS can be relaxed through reflex action alone. This is what happens in defaecation, although filling a balloon in the rectum can induce this relaxation experimentally. Then the fluctuations of potential of the smooth muscle cells of the IAS fall away.

Motility patterns of the EAS

Just like the smooth muscle of the IAS, the striated muscle of the EAS produces potential fluctuations in the resting state, but these increase in amplitude and frequency when a person squeezes. If a person strains, the potential fluctuations of the EAS disappear. The effects of this muscle activity can be manometrically measured. In the resting state the EAS generates a pressure of about 1 kPa (7 mmHg), but during conscious powerful squeezing the EAS can easily produce a pressure of 8 kPa (60 mmHg) or more. During coughing and the Valsalva manoeuvre (deep inspiration followed by vigorous straining with closed glottis) the EAS also contracts, and as a result the rectal contents are retained despite a sudden pressure increase in the abdominal cavity and the rectum. If the rectum is filled with a balloon, the activity in the EAS intensifies.

The rectoanal inhibition reflex

If faeces arrives in the rectum (or if a balloon is blown up in the rectum), the rectum is stretched. The IAS relaxes reflexively, whereas at the same time the EAS contracts involuntarily. This activity can be measured by different techniques:

◆ EMG shows that the fluctuations of the IAS potential fall away, whilst those of the EAS increase in frequency and amplitude.

◆ By manometry it has been established that the pressure in the proximal part of the anal canal (predominantly the IAS) decreases and that the pressure in the distal part (predominantly the EAS) increases.

The relaxation of the IAS that occurs when the rectum is filled is called the rectoanal inhibition reflex. Normally the EAS contracts simultaneously. If the rectum is stretched by a small volume, the relaxation of the IAS is brief (10–20 sec). If stretching is induced by larger volumes (70 ml or more), the IAS relaxes for as long as it is stretched (Figure 95). When the IAS is relaxed, contact is possible between any material in the rectum and the mucosa of the proximal anal canal. It is probably at this point that a person can perceive (through "sampling") that there is gas, liquid or more solid faeces in the rectum. When the IAS has been relaxed for a longer interval, the EAS must be consciously contracted if the rectal contents are to be retained. The rectoanal reflex is activated several times per day without the experience of a defaecation urge. Apparently this reflex frequently occurs unconsciously. But if there are faeces or gas in the rectum, this material stimulates the sensors in the mucosa of the proximal anal canal, at which point sampling occurs.

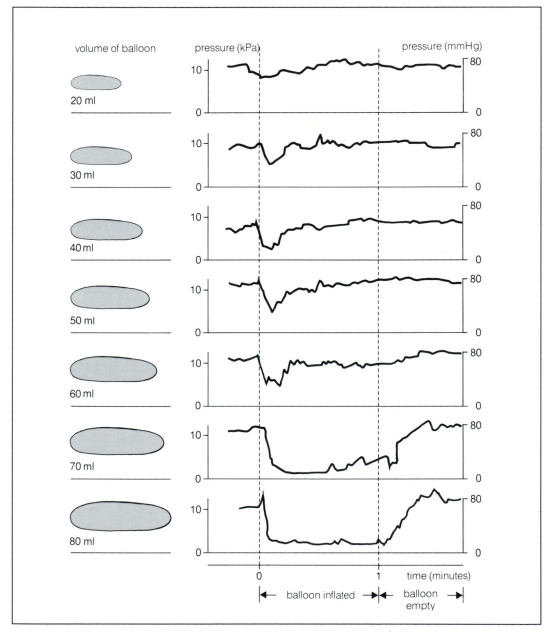

Figure 95: The pressure in the proximal anal canal when the rectum is stretched by a filled balloon for 1 minute. If the rectal stretch is small, the relaxation of the IAS is slight and brief. If this stretch is greater, the IAS relaxes for the whole duration of the stretch. (Reproduced with permission, from Read and Bannister, 1985.)

Defaecation

Relaxation of the IAS and the EAS

If a person feels a defaecation urge, he or she can decide to go to the toilet. The decision to defaecate (immediately) implies physiologically that the person will (immediately) relax the voluntary EAS and the puborectal muscle. At the same time the more lateral muscles of the levator ani muscle contract. This series of events causes the pelvic floor to descend (perineal descent), the anorectal angle to become more obtuse and the muscles of the pelvic floor to form a funnel, as it were, into which the anal canal empties (cf. Figure 96). For

defaecation to occur, the IAS must of course also relax, but this muscle cannot be controlled voluntarily. The IAS always relaxes as a component of the rectoanal inhibition reflex. This rectoanal inhibition reflex can be activated by (involuntary) transport of the faeces from the colon to the rectum, but also through straining*, as a result of which faeces are transported to the rectum.

Defaecation patterns

When the IAS and the EAS are relaxed, some subjects can defaecate without straining. Others have to strain in order to defaecate. Straining is a simultaneous voluntary contraction of the diaphragm and the abdominal muscles. It brings

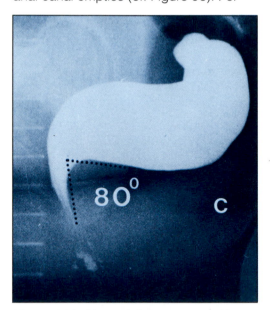

Figure 96A: Normal defaecogram. The subject resists defaecation (by retaining or squeezing). The puborectal muscle is then extra powerfully contracted, as a result of which the anorectal angle is smaller than in the resting state.

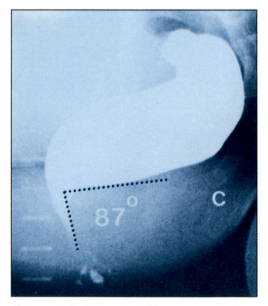

Figure 96B: Normal defaecogram. In the resting state.

* See p. 189 concerning the risks posed by excessively frequent or excessively hard straining.

about an increase in the pressure of the abdominal cavity, which contributes significantly to expelling the faecal bolus. The rectal contractions are weak and do not appear to be propagated. There is wide variation in defaecation, which arises from interpersonal variation and variation in faecal consistency. We shall give here the extreme profiles.

◆ Many persons pass a fairly large quantity of relatively hard stool. They rarely defaecate more than once per day. In these persons defaecation is accompanied by a mass contraction in the left side of the colon. Although this mass contraction can provoke

defaecation, it occurs only after the subject has decided to defaecate.

◆ Some persons pass small quantities of softer stool several times a day. It is possible that this stool is mainly accounted for by the rectal (and distal colonic) contents and that there is no clearly defined mass contraction in the colon.

There are also profiles that fall between these extremes. After defaecation the constriction reflex is activated, with a

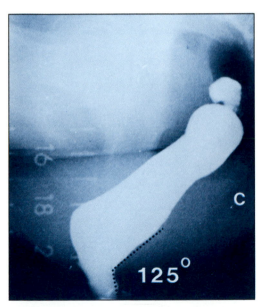

Figure 96C: Normal defaecogram. A healthy volunteer strains and the puborectal muscle and the levator ani muscle relax. As a result the pelvic floor descends and the anorectal angle opens fully out (Reproduced with permission, from Dr R. Goei, Heerlen.)

Intermezzo 24
The anorectal angle

Most of the time the levator ani muscle and the puborectal muscle have a resting tone. As a result the rectum is pulled forward, forming a relatively small angle between the rectal and anal canal (107°, with a deviation of up to 25% on either side) (cf. Figure 96). During squeezing these muscles contract even more and the angle becomes smaller yet (mean size 83°). During defaecation the angle opens fully out (mean size 125°). Much research into defaecation and (in)continence has focused on this angle, which can only be observed by means of defaecography. In a number of persons, however, the rectum and anal canal are positioned in such a way that the angle cannot be measured reliably. The interpersonal variation is substantial and there is a large overlap between the values for healthy subjects and patients.

long-lasting contraction of the EAS and the puborectal muscles. Before long the IAS contracts and the anal canal closes. It is possible that no special stimulus is necessary for these events since the IAS is normally contracted.

If the defaecation urge is resisted

It is also possible (and sometimes desirable) to resist the urge. We should here distinguish between the urge to eliminate faeces and that to eliminate gas.

◆ If the defaecation urge for liquid or more solid faeces is resisted, it subsides "spontaneously". As a component of the defaecation process, a mass contraction can start in the left colon. If the faeces are retained, however, this mass contraction is interrupted (the anocolic reflex). What probably happens here is that the IAS has closed again, the faeces have flowed proximally within the rectum and the rectum has adapted to the new volume (possibly similar to adaptive relaxation of the stomach). A defaecation urge can arise again if additional faeces from the colon reach the rectum or if the faeces are again transported to the anorectal junction by contractions of the rectum. Most persons feel a definite urge if 60–100 ml of faeces is present in the rectum. If the rectum is too full, the defaecation urge is irresistible. In most persons the so-called maximum tolerable volume is 250–400 ml. And even at these volumes the rectal pressure is relatively low (2.5 kPa, 20 mmHg). It is suspected that frequent or long retention leads to disorders in the anorectal region. However, this hypothesis cannot of course be investigated experimentally.

◆ If one resists the urge to expel gas, this urge will also subside within a short time. It is believed that it is not harmful to resist the flatus urge. If this is done the gas is of course resorbed by the intestinal wall and eliminated with exhalation via the blood and lungs.

Intermezzo 25
Relevant questions in the history taking

In order to obtain sufficient information from the patient, it is necessary to put well-directed questions. In this connection it is important that the words used (e.g. "go to the toilet", "bowel movement", "faeces") should be adapted to the patient's world. A rule of thumb is to use the same words that the patient has already used in describing his or her symptoms. Some examples follow.

Constipation
— How often on average do you have a bowel movement per week?
— How often do you have a problem with your bowel movements?
— Is your stool hard or soft?
— Is your stool painful?
— How often per week or per day do you think that you could go to the toilet if you always gave in to the defaecation urge?
— Is there sometimes mucus or blood in your stool? If so, how often?
— Can you tell the difference between stool and gas?
— Do you sometimes have leakage from a loose stool? If so, how often?
— When you have a bowel movement do you have the sensation that not all of the stool has been eliminated?
— Do the people with whom you are in direct contact know that you have this problem?

Incontinence
— How often on average do you have a bowel movement per week?
— How often do you lose stool per week or per day?
— Do you feel it coming and are you then unable to stop it?
— Do you feel it only after it's too late?
— Do you sometimes find it difficult to defaecate and if so how often?
— Is your stool soft or hard?
— Is your stool thin or fairly thick?
— Are your bowel movements painful?
— How often per week or per day do you feel that you could go to the toilet if you always gave in to the defaecation urge?
— Is there also sometimes mucus or blood in your stool? If so, how often?
— Can you tell the difference between stool and gas?
— When you have a bowel movement do you have the feeling that not all the stool has been eliminated?
— What do you do so that your problem will give you as little trouble as possible?
— Do the people with whom you are in direct contact know that you have this problem?

Motility disturbances of the anorectum and pelvic floor

An obstacle

Before patients with these disturbances can be optimally treated, a thorny obstacle must be overcome: **the patient's embarrassment**. Patients with incontinence are notorious for being so ashamed of their problem that they repeatedly put off going to a doctor and once they do go, they give only vague and incomplete information. These patients are generally afraid that the outside world will find out about their problem since this disorder is difficult to hide. Because of the shame it is especially difficult to live with. Many of these patients are ashamed even before a doctor; sometimes they do not spontaneously mention their symptoms. The best approach for the doctor is to put a number of directed questions by way of obtaining a picture that is as close to complete as possible (Intermezzo 25, p. 187). In addition, it is sometimes desirable to record an actual defaecation for examination purposes. However, a number of patients are not able to defaecate in an unfamiliar environment. (This inability is not necessarily a defaecation disorder.) In some countries there are patients' support groups which can help patients get over severe embarrassment.

A relationship between constipation, incontinence and pain

The most frequent symptoms of motility disturbances of the pelvic floor are as follows: constipation, faecal incontinence, pain in the lower abdomen, perianal or anorectal pain and incomplete defaecation even after hard straining. Although constipation and incontinence would seem to exclude one another, constipation can lead indirectly to incontinence.

◆ Many patients with constipation strain repeatedly for a long time in an attempt to defaecate. This habit leads secondarily to damage to the mucosa, the sacral nerves and the muscles of the pelvic floor. This damage can induce faecal incontinence.

◆ Constipation is often accompanied by impaction, i.e. the accumulation of hard faecal material in the colon, sigmoid colon and rectum. Fluid faeces can flow past this faecaloma and leak out through the anal canal ("overflow incontinence" diarrhoea resulting from constipation or impaction is called paradoxical diarrhoea).

Figure 97 gives an overview of the plausible causal relationships, but not all of them have been shown to be important. What stands out in this scheme is that prolonged hard straining in constipation can bring about severe nerve and muscle damage. The consequences of this damage are often more serious than the constipation itself. It is important to ensure that the patient does not strain too much by treating the constipation and explaining his or her condition properly.

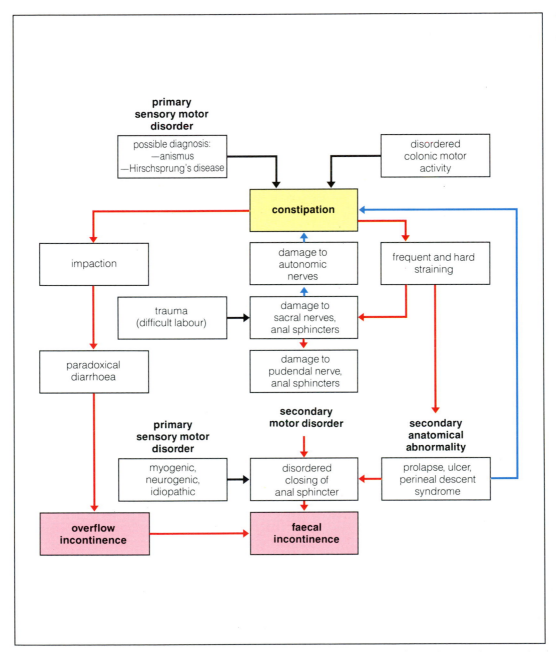

Figure 97: Schematic overview of the causes of constipation and faecal incontinence. It can be seen here that constipation can secondarily provoke faecal incontinence. Some of these connections are still hypothetical.

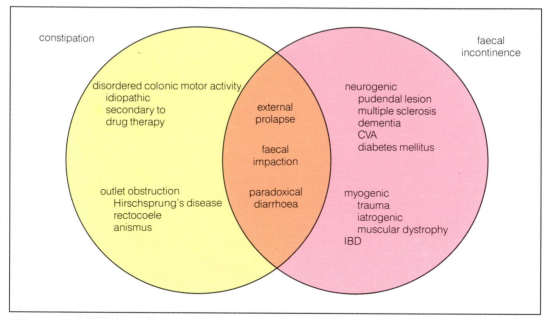

Figure 98: Overview of the most important disorders that can bring about constipation, faecal incontinence or both.

Pain and constipation can be related. Defaecation can be attended by pain in, amongst other disorders, rectal ulcer, tumour, fissure or intussusception. A number of patients react to pain by a reflexive constriction of the anal canal. Although all these symptoms are related to one another and occur together, we can discuss them more informatively if we deal with them separately. Figure 98 gives a brief overview of the disorders or conditions that accompany constipation and/or faecal incontinence.

Anorectal constipation

By means of good history taking, physical examination, sigmoidoscopy and, when appropriate, anal endosonography, in about 80% of patients a disorder can be identified that has (probably) induced the constipation. A diagnostic flow chart (Figure 111, p. 234) indicates the factors which can be focused on as well as the relevant examinations and when they should be performed.

The symptoms
Healthy volunteers sometimes also have difficulty defaecating or defaecate incompletely. But if, in particular, a person finds it necessary to strain at more than one in four defaecations and if this occurs more than twice a week, the constipation warrants further attention. An anorectal examination is justified in the following situations:
— when a patient frequently finds it necessary to strain hard when attempting to defaecate;
— when a patient has the feeling of an obstructed defaecation;
— when a patient has the feeling that only part of the faeces have been expelled.
So that an impression can be obtained of the (conscious) anorectal sensitivity, the patient is asked if he feels that he is able to go to the toilet and if he needs to do this urgently. The patient should also be asked if there is any mucus or blood in the faeces. If so, there may be a prolapse, a solitary rectal ulcer, inflammatory bowel disease (IBD) or a tumour.

Diagnostic examination

Colon or anorectum and pelvic floor?
It should first be attempted to determine whether the symptoms can be attributed to delayed colonic transit or a pelvic floor disorder (Figure 111, p. 234). In most patients there is delayed colonic transit (p. 158). In some patients the physical examination already provides strong evidence of pelvic floor disorders (e.g. anatomical abnormalities or faeces in the rectum).
◆ If a patient seldom feels a defaecation urge, delayed colonic transit can be envisaged.
◆ On the other hand, persons who regularly feel a defaecation urge but who cannot defaecate are likely to have a pelvic floor disorder.
◆ There is a third group of patients, however, who have diminished sensitivity in the anorectal zone and therefore rarely feel a defaecation urge.
Finally, in some patients it is not possible to differentiate clearly between a disorder of the colon and a disorder of the anorectal region.

Motility disturbance or anatomical abnormality?
If the patient has a (probable) pelvic floor disorder the crucial question is whether this disorder arises primarily from a motility disturbance or an anatomical abnormality. The latter, however, can also result from a motility disturbance (Figure 97). This means that the constipation is not automatically cleared up by correction of the abnormality. A number of anatomical abnormalities can

be detected by physical examination and sigmoidoscopy (prolapse, fissure, tumour). Digital anal examination can reveal a palpable prolapse. Other anatomical abnormalities, however, come to light only at defaecography. If the patient is asked to strain while sitting on the toilet, it can be seen whether a prolapse consists of mucosa alone or mucosa *and* muscle tissue. When the patient strains, normally the pelvic floor descends (perineal descent); when it descends more than 2 cm, one speaks of a pathological perineal descent. A special device (a perineometer) has been developed for measuring the perineal descent during straining. To identify positively motility disorders of the pelvic floor, anorectal manometry, EMG or defaecography is necessary.

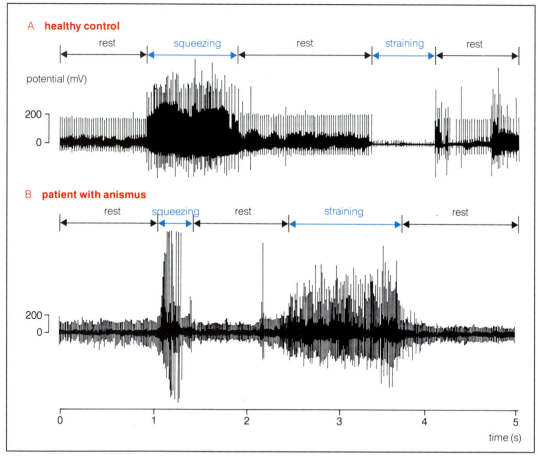

Figure 99: An electromyogram of the puborectal muscle. A: Normal: during squeezing the activity increases and during straining it is almost absent. B: A patient with anismus: during squeezing and during straining the activity increases. (Reproduced with permission, from Swash and Snooks, 1985.)

Often a combination of these techniques is used.

Functional outlet obstructions

Because of various factors, faecal transit through the rectum and anal canal can be impeded in a condition called anorectal "outlet obstruction". The outlet obstruction can be due to defective motility of the anal sphincters or the pelvic floor muscles ("functional outlet obstruction") or of an anatomical abnormality ("anatomical outlet obstruction"). Only if the muscles of the anal sphincter and the pelvic floor undergo well-co-ordinated contractions can the faeces pass easily. Otherwise faecal passage through the anal canal is extremely difficult. (It could be compared to trying to squeeze a tube of toothpaste empty with the cap screwed on.)

Anismus

In a number of patients with constipation it has been found that during straining the EAS and also the puborectal muscle and levator ani do not relax. In some patients a paradoxical contraction of these muscles has even been observed during straining (Figure 99). If the puborectal muscle and/or levator ani do not relax, the pelvic floor does not descend and the rectoanal angle decreases rather than becoming obtuse. This disorder can clearly be observed by means of defaecography (Figure 100). It is called anismus and it is a chronic defaecation disorder. It is an acquired dysfunction and can begin at any age. Often psychological factors also appear to play a role. Patients with anismus have great difficulty starting the defaecation process. Even if they do

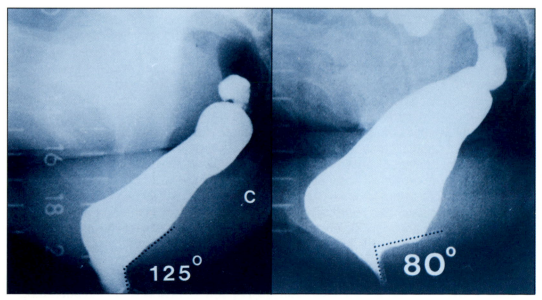

Figure 100: Defaecograms recorded during straining. A: A healthy volunteer. B: A patient with anismus. During straining the puborectal muscle remains contracted, so that the anorectal angle remains acute (Reproduced with permission, from Dr R. Goei, Heerlen.)

manage to produce faeces, generally they are not able to fully empty the rectum. Often the picture is characterized by laxative abuse and impaction, overflow incontinence and rectal pain. A diagnosis of anismus can be made after defaecography, the expulsion test, manometry or EMG during defaecation.

Treatment. In the past it was attempted to treat anismus by totally or partially transecting the puborectal muscle or the EAS. The results, however, were disappointing and these operations are no longer performed. Now training through biofeedback appears to be promising. (See Intermezzo 28, p. 208.).

Hirschsprung's disease

Hirschsprung's disease is the first thoroughly investigated motility disorder that leads to constipation. This disease is congenital and is characterized by the absence of nerve cells in the ENS in the rectum. The segment of the rectum lacking nerve cells can be small or extensive and it can lie proximally on the junction between sigmoid colon and rectum or more distally, even as far as the anorectal junction. The part of the rectum without ganglia can act as a functional stenosis; faeces accumulate proximally and the proximal intestine (rectum or sigmoid colon) becomes dilated. The more extensive the region without nerve cells, the more severe the symptoms. It is typical of Hirschsprung's disease that the rectoanal inhibition reflex is either significantly diminished or absent. Anorectal manometry is an important technique in making the diagnosis; if the rectoanal inhibition reflex is present, Hirschsprung's

disease is eliminated; if this reflex is absent (Figure 101), the diagnosis should be confirmed histologically by rectal biopsies stained for acetylcholinesterase. In Hirschsprung's disease, despite the absence of ganglia, an increase in the number of nerve fibres is often observed. In some patients, however, there are no nerve cells nor nerve fibres at all. In classical Hirschsprung's disease, severe constipation is observed even in babies. It is believed that a number of adult patients with an outlet obstruction have an "adult Hirschsprung's disease" disorder. It is thought that a short segment of the rectum at the anorectal junction contains a substantially reduced number of nerve cells. Because this aganglionic segment is short and located distally, the symptoms would be expected to manifest themselves only at a later age. Nevertheless, it is very difficult to make the diagnosis "adult Hirschsprung's". Here too anorectal manometry and acetylcholinesterase staining are important. The answer to the question of whether this abnormality actually exists is not yet clear, however; it is well known, for example, that there is great variation in the number of nerve cells in the ENS of this part of the rectum in normal persons.

Treatment. In (classical) Hirschsprung's disease the aganglionic and dilated intestinal segment is resected, whilst the IAS and EAS remain in *situ* (Duhamel or Soave procedure). The surgical result is excellent, although in some patients a myectomy of the IAS is still necessary. In contrast, in the past, in adult Hirschsprung's disease myectomy of the IAS and a resection of the affected

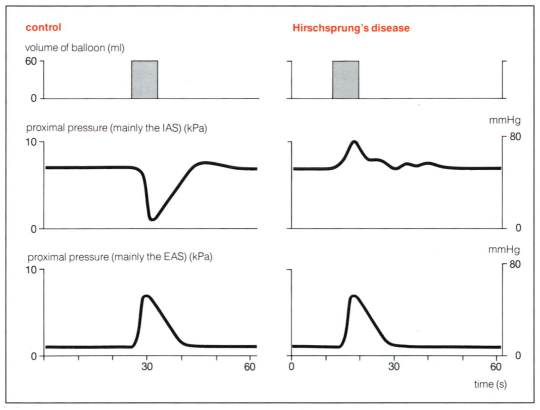

Figure 101: Manometric recording of the rectoanal inhibition reflex. A: Normal. B: Patient with Hirschsprung's disease: the rectoanal inhibition reflex is absent. To make the diagnosis, however, a biopsy of the rectum is still necessary.

segment were performed, but the results were variable.

Disordered anorectal sensitivity

In some patients the sensitivity of the rectum and the anorectal zone is disturbed: the sensitivity is excessive or insufficient. Two forms of the condition are distinguished in patients with **hyposensitivity** of the anorectal region.

◆ A diminished **conscious** sensitivity. These patients either feel no defaecation urge or feel one only when the rectum is copiously filled,

and often they cannot discriminate or they can discriminate only subnormally between the presence of faeces or gas above the anal canal. The rectoanal inhibition reflex is intact however. This picture occurs after an **acute transverse cord lesion** or after other lesions of the ascending nerves (e.g. in **diabetes mellitus**) or brain lesions (CVA).

◆ A diminished **unconscious** sensitivity. These patients show either no rectoanal inhibition reflex or a diminution of this reflex, although they experience a defaecation urge and often can distinguish between gas and faeces. Here damage to or degeneration of the ENS is involved.

◆ This profile occurs in **Hirschsprung's disease**. Also, in some patients the IAS relaxes but the EAS does not contract. This pattern is observed if, amongst other disorders, there is **damage to the pudendal nerve**. Incontinence can be the result.

In some patients the total anorectal sensitivity (conscious and unconscious) has been lost. Disturbances of the conscious and unconscious sensitivity of the rectum can be quantified by gradually filling a balloon in the rectum and simultaneously measuring the pressure, or by electrical stimulation with a constant current. By using the balloon, the volume to which the patient is sensitive and at which the inhibition reflex occurs is registered. It is suggested that in some patients prolonged, excessively hard straining has damaged the nerve cells. A primary effect of this hyposensitivity is constipation. In a number of patients secondary incontinence is the result. **Hypersensitivity** is also observed, in IBS patients amongst others. In these patients, if a small volume (sometimes 10 ml) of faeces arrives in the rectum, a slight urge is felt. However, they are not able to expel this small volume, so that the urge continues to be felt.

Anatomical anomalies of the anorectum

There are several variants of anatomical abnormalities in the anorectum which cause the formation of an outlet

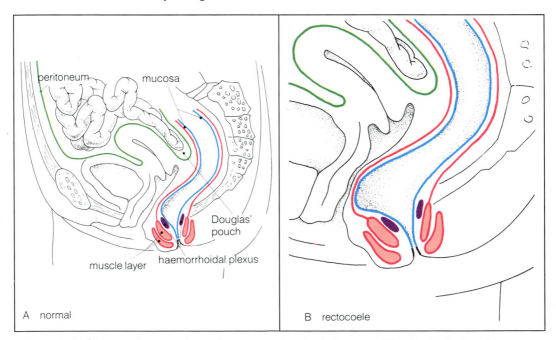

Figure 102: Schematic overview of some anatomical abnormalities that can lead to anorectal constipation. A: Normal. B: Rectocoele.

obstruction, induce incontinence or are present without provoking symptoms.

Rectocoele

Prolapse of the rectum is found mainly in women. It generally protrudes ventrally into the vagina wall (Figure 102B), which can render defaecation difficult. Small rectocoeles are common and do not require an operation. If the rectocoele is larger, surgical reconstruction of the ventral wall should be considered. Patients with a large rectocoele can sometimes reduce it with their fingers from the vagina to the point where they can defaecate. If this digital correction works reasonably well, it is shown that the defaecation mechanism is still intact. If it is, the chance of the patient's being

able to defaecate normally after surgical repair of the ventral wall is maximal.

Enterocoele

A loop of the small intestine can compress the rectum when a person strains. This can happen when a loop of the small intestine protrudes through an opening in the peritoneal membrane. But generally the peritoneal membrane protrudes too far toward the pelvic floor (because Douglas' pouch is too deep) and an intestinal loop falls down into it (Figure 102C). This intestinal loop can cause an outlet obstruction. For patients with this disorder the opening in the peritoneal membrane can be repaired or Douglas' pouch can be reduced. The symptoms will then be significantly reduced.

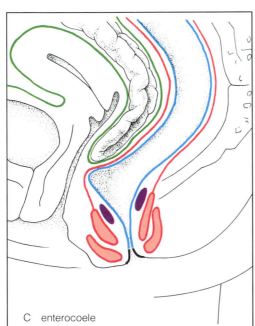

C   enterocoele

Figure 102C: Enterocoele caused by a pathologically deep Douglas' pouch.

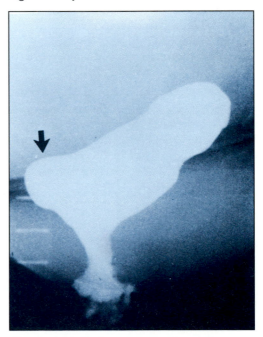

Figure 103: Defaecogram of a patient with a rectocoele. (Reproduced with permission, from Dr R. Goei, Heerlen.)

Prolapses and haemorrhoids

A portion of the rectal wall can protrude. Sometimes only the mucosa protrudes (mucosal prolapse), sometimes the mucosa and the haemorrhoidal plexus and sometimes the mucosa and the muscularis protrudes (complete prolapse, Table 8). If an entire segment of an intestine protrudes, the abnormality is called an intussusception (Figure 104C). Sometimes the protrusion remains limited to the rectum (internal or occult prolapse), sometimes it remains limited to the interior of the anal canal and sometimes it extends to outside the anal canal. The last abnormality is referred to as an external prolapse (Figure 104D) or external haemorrhoids (piles).

Complications. One in five patients with an internal prolapse develops an external prolapse (Table 8). There is a risk that the top of an internal prolapse or intussusception will become strangulated (especially when the patient strains), with ischaemia as a possible consequence. A **solitary rectal ulcer** may then form, almost always at the top of the prolapse. Complications of a prolapse (and haemorrhoids) are **constipation** and/or **incontinence**. An external prolapse is more serious than an internal prolapse: about 30% of patients with an internal prolapse and about 50% with an external prolapse are incontinent. The question arises whether the outlet obstruction is caused by the prolapse or vice versa. It is believed that generally the outlet obstruction is primary; it leads to excessive straining, which could in turn induce prolapse. Patients with a rectal prolapse can become incontinent in the long term as a result of nerve damage. The prolapse by itself does not produce incontinence, but nerve damage does.

What prolapses?	into the rectum	into the anal canal	past the anal canal
only the mucosa	internal mucosal prolapse	anal mucosal prolapse	external mucosal prolapse
mucosa plus haemorrhoidal plexus		internal haemorrhoids	external haemorrhoids
mucosa plus muscularis (non-circular)	internal complete prolapse	anal complete prolapse	external complete prolapse
mucosa plus muscularis (circular)	internal intussusception	anal intussusception	external intussusception

Table 8: The relationship between the different forms of prolapses and haemorrhoids. The arrows indicate which variants can arise from which. Hypothetical transformations are indicated with a broken line and an arrow.

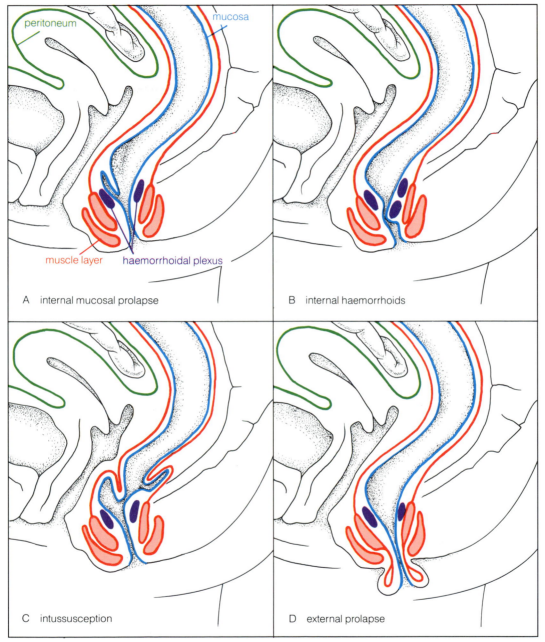

Figure 104: Schematic overview of some anatomical abnormalities that can lead to constipation. A: Internal mucosal prolapse; B: Internal haemorrhoids; C: Intussusception of the proximal rectum into the distal rectum. D: External prolapse.

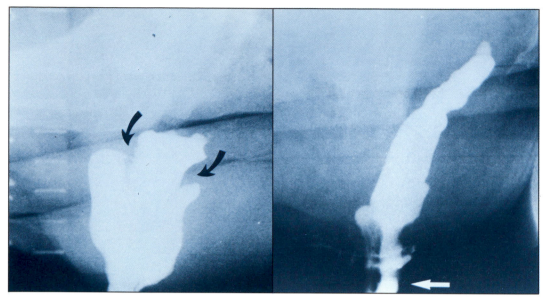

Figure 105: Defaecograms. Left: Circular intussusception of the proximal rectum into the distal rectum. Right: Mucosal prolapse. (Reproduced with permission, from Dr R. Goei, Heerlen.)

Treatment. A **mucosal prolapse** is successfully treated with rubber band ligation. The surgical treatment of an **internal (complete) prolapse**, however, is controversial. Good results have been reported for rectopexy in patients with a solitary rectal ulcer and an outlet obstruction. **Haemorrhoids** can be treated effectively with rubber band ligation and electro or infrared coagulation and in some cases by haemorrhoidectomy. Of all the anorectal abnormalities the **external prolapse** can be best treated surgically. Rectopexy is the operation of choice. In this operation the rectum is entirely mobilized and fixed to the sacrum. By means of this operation the anatomical abnormality can be corrected but that does not automatically imply that the incontinence or constipation will cease. About half of the patients with an external prolapse and incontinence regain their continence after the operation. If the anatomical abnormality is corrected, their anal sphincter is again able to constrict the anus adequately. However, patients with a pre-operative constipation and a prolapse almost invariably still have the constipation after the operation, and sometimes the condition is even more serious. This observation is in line with the view that a prolapse is generally not a cause of constipation. In older patients for whom abdominal surgery is contra-indicated, the operation after Delorme's method should be performed (Watts et al., 1985).

Intermezzo 26
The terminology

Many concepts having to do with disorders in the anorectal region are not to be found in medical dictionaries. Therefore we shall here give a brief description of the most important ones.

◆ **Anismus**: a disorder in which the EAS or the puborectal muscle or the levator ani fail to relax during defaecation, and remain contracted or even contract more powerfully (also called the spastic pelvic floor syndrome).

◆ **Enterocoele**: prolapse of a loop of the small intestine into either a pathologically deep Douglas' pouch (Figure 102C) or into an opening in the peritoneal membrane.

◆ **Impaction (faecal)**: the presence of relatively hard faeces in the colon or rectum. The faeces are as solid as putty or even harder.

◆ **Incontinence (faecal)**: a disorder in which the patient cannot retain faeces or gas.

◆ **Intussusception (= invagination)**: prolapse of a part of an intestine into an immediately adjoining part.

◆ **Outlet obstruction**: umbrella term for all those disorders in which anal transit is impeded by anatomical anomalies or inappropriate movements of muscles of the anus or pelvic floor. Consequently, a distinction is made between functional and anatomic outlet obstruction.

◆ **Paradoxical diarrhoea**: false diarrhoea: diarrhoea caused by constipation or impaction.

◆ **Perineal descent**: of the pelvic floor during defaecation.

◆ **Perineal descent syndrome**: umbrella term for disorders that are accompanied by an excessive sinking of the pelvic floor during straining.

◆ **Procidentia**: prolapse

◆ **Prolapse**: protrusion of the rectal mucosa or rectal wall. Several variants are distinguished (Table 8 and Figure 104), depending on whether only the mucosa or the mucosa and the muscularis protrude, and depending on how far these structures protrude (into the rectum itself, into the anal canal or past the anal canal). It is advisable with prolapse always to specify what has protruded (mucosal, complete or haemorrhoids) and into what it has sunk (internal = occult, anal or external). If the whole rectal wall protrudes circularly, the term used is intussusception (Figure 104C).

◆ **Rectocoele**: prolapse of the rectum; almost invariably the prolapse is into the vagina (Figure 102A).

◆ **Solitary rectal ulcer**: ulcer in the rectum, generally at the top of an internal prolapse or intussusception.

Megarectum

Patients with a megarectum feel a defaecation urge only if a large volume of faeces is present. The faeces reside for a long time in the rectum and dry out. Only with great difficulty can the patient expel the large volume of faeces from the oversized rectum. Megarectum is sometimes congenital and sometimes acquired. Since conservative measures are ineffective, the choice falls upon a resection of the rectum with a colo-anal anastomosis (the Duhamel procedure). However, this technique yields only moderately successful results.

Anal stenosis

The anal canal can be narrowed by prolapses, fistulas, abscesses and fissures. Anal strictures can be treated effectively by means of myotomy of the IAS with or without dilation of the anus by means of anusoplasty.

Incontinence

With most incontinent patients a reasonable understanding of the disorder can now be achieved by means of a good history taking, a physical examination and anal endosonography. In a number of cases it is appropriate to perform manometry or an EMG so that muscle and nerve disorders can be differentiated from one another. If the indication is accurate, there is a fairly good chance that treatment will succeed.

The symptoms

Faecal incontinence is defined as the loss of control of the retention of liquid, gas and solid intestinal contents. A distinction is made between a mild and a severe form. In **mild** incontinence the patient's underwear is occasionally slightly soiled and sometimes there is loss of control of flatus and liquid faeces. This type of (overflow) incontinence often occurs in connection with impaction or surgical damage to the IAS. Mild incontinence occurs fairly frequently in older persons with diminished rectal sensitivity. Many IBS patients also complain of mild incontinence. The great majority of these patients report that they have diarrhoea. Patients with **severe** incontinence suffer from uncontrolled loss of formed faeces. The faeces can be lost sporadically (e.g. once a week) or very frequently (several times per day). Some patients make it a point of familiarizing themselves with all the toilets in department stores and along the motorway so that they can reach them quickly. If a patient can still get about easily or has easy access to a toilet in the neighbourhood, his or her incontinence often poses less of a problem. In the severe forms of incontinence, generally there is impairment of the puborectal muscle, the IAS and the EAS. Most of these patients have a low resting pressure in the anal canal and can build up almost no pressure during squeezing. This profile indicates neuropathy. When the rectal pressure rises above the anal canal pressure incontinence is the result.

Diagnostic examination

As with other disorders, with incontinence the obvious causes should be focused on first: dementia, CVA or a trauma (whether or not consequent upon difficult labour). When the incontinence is accompanied by constipation, one's attention should first be directed to this, because when constipation is reduced, the incontinence often subsides. Supplementary examinations should be directed to the detection of **anatomical abnormalities** (e.g. external prolapse). Then one should try, as far as is possible, to differentiate **myogenic and neurogenic incontinence** (Table 11, p. 224). By physical examination, damage to the sphincter is often disclosed. Digital anal examination gives an indication of the sphincter tone, the squeeze pressure, any asymmetry of the sphincter, a global impression of the puborectal muscle tone and the presence of a palpable occult prolapse. A diminished or an asymmetrical anal sphincter tension can point to muscle damage or an innervation dysfunction. Anal endosonography is an excellent method of detecting damage to the anal sphincters. Sigmoidoscopy is also useful in pinpointing anatomical anomalies.

In some patients there is strong evidence of neurogenic incontinence (e.g. CVA, dementia, multiple sclerosis or diabetes mellitus). It is much more difficult to identify conclusively lesions of the pudendal nerve (this is possible only in a few centres where an EMG is done of individual muscle fibres and the conduction velocity of the pudendal nerve measured) (Figure 106). In many patients with the so-called "idiopathic incontinence" pudendal nerve dysfunction can be detected by means of a special examination. It then becomes clear that they have neurogenic incontinence.

Myogenic incontinence
A frequent cause of incontinence is impairment or tearing of the anal sphincters, for example, as a result of difficult labour, impalement, anal rape or anal surgery. A muscular disorder (e.g. muscular dystrophy) can also provoke myogenic incontinence.

Treatment. If the muscle damage can be accurately located, surgical repair is often successful. (More than 80% of patients regain their continence after surgery.) The muscle stumps are placed (in overlapping fashion) over and sutured to one another, possibly in combination with a reconstruction of the anterior part of the perineum.

Neurogenic incontinence
The other important cause of incontinence is degeneration of or damage to the nerves. In some patients there is a brain disorder (in dementia or CVA). In addition, there may be damage to or degeneration of the pudendal nerve (e.g. in diabetes mellitus or multiple sclerosis). Signs of neurogenic incontinence can be disclosed by an EMG study (Table 11, p. 224).

Treatment. In neurogenic incontinence, sphincteroplasty is less successful. If no lesion of the sphincter can be found in these patients, a post-anal repair can be performed (Henry and Thomson 1985). About 60% of patients benefit from this operation but only 20–50% regain full continence of flatus and liquid and solid stool. With a weak sphincter it is sometimes possible to regain some continence by means of sphincter training (Intermezzo 28, p. 208). If all surgical and conservative measures fail, the only other possibility is to create a stoma or anus praeternaturalis (AP).

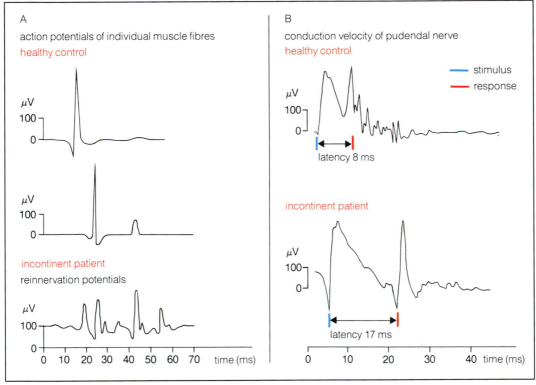

Figure 106: In order to establish that a neurogenic incontinence is due to a disordered pudendal nerve it is necessary to perform an EMG. By means of this test various neurogenic disturbances can be identified. A: Conduction of individual muscle fibres: in healthy volunteers one or two peaks occur, but in the incontinent patient there are several peaks (reinnervation potentials), which indicates that there is a nerve lesion. B: Measurement of the conduction velocity of the pudendal nerve. This nerve is electrically stimulated and the response of the EAS is recorded. The normal latency is about 8 ms. If there is degeneration of the pudendal nerve, the latency can be much greater.

Incontinence of liquid faeces

Some patients suffer incontinence of liquid but not of solid faeces. Most of these patients are elderly (often inoperable) and have diminished sensitivity of the rectum and in some cases a megarectum. A number of them also have an impaction. They might benefit from induced defaecation early in the morning (by means of a laxative or enema) and then suppression of diarrhoea during the day by taking loperamide.

Chronic perianal or anorectal pain

In most patients with perianal or anorectal pain the cause of the pain (anal fistulas and intersphincteric abscess, thrombosed haemorrhoids and anorectal carcinoma) can be established and treated. In addition, some perianal and anorectal pain syndromes have been described that may be attributable to disorders of the anorectum or pelvic floor.

Coccygodynia

Coccygodynia is a disorder marked by vague, piercing pain in the region of the sacrum and the coccyx and in the surrounding muscles and other soft tissues. It is accompanied by rectal and perianal nagging pain that sometimes radiates to the thighs and buttocks. Patients report that sitting provokes or exacerbates the pain. Most of these patients are women, the symptoms generally develop between age 50 and 60 years, and the pain often persists for years. The cause is unknown.

Proctalgia fugax

The cause of proctalgia fugax is also unknown. It begins suddenly with vague pain that quickly intensifies, sometimes becoming severe and crampy and lasting for about 30 minutes. The pain is always felt in a well-defined place in the anal canal or in the lower part of the rectum, just above the EAS. The pain attacks occur mostly at night, but sometimes during the day. Proctalgia fugax is more frequent in men than in women. It often begins in young adults and falls away spontaneously in mid-life. Sometimes sitting on the floor, stretching the legs upward and drawing them as closely as possible toward the belly reduces the pain. It is believed that the syndrome arises from crampy, spastic contractions of the rectum or of the muscles of the pelvic floor, for which reason it is often called the "levator syndrome". It occurs more frequently in IBS patients.

Pain in pathological perineal descent

In patients with pathological perineal descent, pain sometimes occurs in the perineum. The pain arises during straining when the perineum falls excessively. It persists after defaecation, occurs when the patient has been standing or walking for a long time and often subsides when he or she lies down. The symptoms sometimes decrease when defaecation improves.

Hypertrophy of the IAS

A characteristic disorder has recently been found by means of endosonography in a number of patients from the same family with idiopathic anal pain. These patients have a hypertrophic IAS with pain that occurs mainly at night. Lateral sphincterotomy has been found to reduce their pain substantially.

Idiopathic perianal pain

Finally, there is a group of patients with a poorly described anal and perianal pain—the "chronic idiopathic perianal pain". It is a continuous, nagging and burning pain in the anal canal that occurs late in the day. It can radiate to the lower abdomen, the thighs, the perineum and the vagina. Often these patients have undergone spinal surgery. It is suspected that psychiatric disturbances also play a role in this pathology.

Treatment of perianal or anorectal pain

If no cause can be discovered, the treatment of perianal or anorectal pain is extremely difficult, so that many of these patients go from one doctor to another. In fact only hypertrophy of the IAS responds well to treatment. Patients with anal and perianal pain are often treated with antidepressants, but with little success. Surgery does not help. Analgesics (NSAID) sometimes reduce the pain to some extent.

Intermezzo 27
The perineal descent syndrome

During a normal defaecation the pelvic floor sinks slightly. (A descent of 2 cm is normal.) In a number of patients, however, the pelvic floor sinks too far when the patient defaecates (or strains). This pathology is referred to as the perineal descent syndrome. In fact it is not a distinct disorder but a complication that is sometimes accompanied by symptoms of other anatomical anomalies. Excessive perineal descent is generally the consequence of weak pelvic floor muscles. This weakness can arise from neuronal degeneration or damage, old age, difficult labour or chronic, excessive, prolonged straining in constipation or from a combination of these factors. Patients with the perineal descent syndrome have a long history of excessive straining at stool. An early complication of an abnormal perineal descent is constipation; a late complication is incontinence, when the innervation of both the IAS and the EAS is disordered. The perineal descent syndrome itself is not treatable, but any accompanying complications (e.g. prolapse or incontinence) can be treated as they would be if they occurred alone.

Intermezzo 28
Biofeedback training

Biofeedback refers to a technique in which a person for whom a physiological recording is done can immediately observe (either visually or auditively) the results. Any type of biological information can be recorded, e.g. an EMG of the EAS, manometry of the anal canal, an ECG, an EEG, etc. By means of the observation a person can try to modify systematically a parameter in what is called biofeedback training. Often the person does not know how to do this, but learns to do so by trial and error. Biofeedback training is supervised by a physiotherapist, who does his or her best to motivate the patient and encourages each step forward, however small. This technique is used for patients with anismus and some forms of incontinence.

◆ **Anismus**. The activity of the EAS is recorded (by EMG or manometry) and the patient is shown the trace on a screen. The patient can then see a resting EAS activity when he relaxes and an increased activity on squeezing the EAS. At the start of training the patient sees that when he strains, the EAS activity also increases, whereas it should do just the opposite. Subsequently the patient is instructed to lower the level of activity while he strains. In biofeedback training for anismus it is important that the patient should be very motivated and that he should not have any acute psychological problems.

◆ **Incontinence**. In patients with neurogenic incontinence who still have some innervation of the EAS, biofeedback training can be useful. The EAS activity is also displayed to them (by EMG or manometry). A balloon is inserted into the patient's rectum and blown up (volume about 60 ml). In this way the inhibition reflex is stimulated and if it is intact, the patient feels this filling of the rectum. The patient is instructed to try to raise the activity level of the EAS. As a result of this training, the muscle strength of the EAS can increase as can the sensitivity of the rectum. The latter factor is also important for continence. An important condition in biofeedback training in neurogenic incontinence is that there should be at least some perception of rectal filling and at least some innervation of the EAS. In overflow and idiopathic incontinence the results are disappointing. It is also sometimes useful for patients who can contract their EAS to do power training of the EAS (without biofeedback) by squeezing the sphincter several times per day.

To be effective, biofeedback training requires multiple sessions (e.g. 25). After successful training patients with anismus can defaecate without much problem and incontinent patients regain their continence. This improvement can become permanent; success rates of up to 70% have been reported.

Conclusion

The retention of faeces and gas on the one hand and defaecation on the other are complex processes. They require that several groups of smooth and striated muscles should contract and relax in a highly co-ordinated fashion. Primarily by means of manometry, defaecography and EMG, it has been possible to gather solid scientific data on this subject.

Motility or anatomical abnormalities of the rectum, anus and pelvic floor can provoke constipation or incontinence. However, precious little is known about the actual causes of anorectal and pelvic floor syndromes. In fact it has been shown only that limited muscle and nerve damage (as a result of partus, spearing or surgery) can provoke symptoms. But apparently the same lesions can give rise to different complaints. It is believed that a defective co-ordination between the different muscles may be the manifestation of an acquired defective reaction or it may be psychogenic. The different abnormalities and symptoms are so interwoven that no-one to date has been able to sort them out.

Notwithstanding, anorectal and pelvic floor studies are assuming an increasingly important role in the evaluation of the patient's symptoms. Undoubtedly it will be possible to disentangle further anorectal and pelvic floor syndromes in the future by means of physiological studies. Physiological tests already permit a choice of treatment.

In recent years a better determination of indications has improved surgical treatment, although much research remains to be done into the causes of anorectal and pelvic floor syndromes.

References

Felt-Bersma, RJF, Clinical indications for anorectal function investigations. Scand J Gastroenterol 1990; 25 (suppl 178): 1–6.

Goei R. Defecography. A radiological study on anorectal function and related disorders. Rijksunversiteit Limburg 1990.

Henry MM, Thomson JPS Treatment: (i) Postanal repair. In: Henry MM, Swash M, eds. Coloproctology and the pelvic floor. London: Butterworth 1985: 228–234

Read NW, Bannister JJ. Anorectal manometry: techniques in health and anorectal disease. In: Henry MM, Swash M, eds. Coloproctology and the pelvic floor. London: Butterworth 1985: 65–87

Swash M, Snooks SJ. Electromyography in pelvic floor disorders. In: Henry MM, Swash M, eds. Coloproctology and the pelvic floor. London: Butterworth 1985: 88–103

Watts JD, Rothenberger DA, Goldberg SM. Treatment. In: Henry MM, Swash M, eds. Coloproctology and the pelvic floor. London: Butterworth 1985: 308–339

Diagnosis

Chapter 12

From symptom to diagnosis

In this chapter the most important symptoms that accompany motility disorders of the digestive tract will be reviewed. For each symptom we provide an overview of the diseases that should be suspected and the manner in which the diagnosis can be made.

Introduction

Suppose you are examining a patient
with symptoms that point to dysmotility
of the digestive tract but that could also
have a completely different cause. The
art here consists in making a diagnosis
as efficiently as possible and in such a
way that other life-threatening or
treatable diseases are excluded with
sufficient confidence. In this chapter we
shall provide guidelines in this respect:
— what diseases can these symptoms
  point to?
— how can you efficiently identify or
  exclude these?
We shall provide a diagnostic flow chart
for each symptom or symptom complex.
In principle it is possible to use this while
one makes a diagnosis. Generally,
however, these flow charts are used as
a memory aid by way of checking
whether one has thought of the most
important diagnostic alternatives and
investigation techniques.

In this chapter our point of departure is
the individual symptom. In practice
many patients suffer from several
symptoms. Nevertheless, most patients
present with a main symptom. In spite of
this limitation, we anticipate that the
reader will find the overview useful.

Dyspeptic symptoms

Dyspeptic symptoms (amongst others pain in the upper abdomen, nausea, vomiting and abdominal fullness) are addressed here together, because they often accompany one another. Various disorders attend a delayed or an accelerated gastric emptying (see Tables 9 and 10, pp. 220 and 221); the dysmotility can provoke dyspepsia. The examination should at first be geared to excluding various situations or disorders (Figure 109, p. 230), of which the most frequent follow:
— infections and inflammations of the gastrointestinal tract,
— organic abnormalities outside the stomach (gall stones, pancreatitis, pancreatic carcinoma, colonic carcinoma),
— constipation, IBS,
— metabolic disorders,
— hormonal disorders (hypo- or hyperthyroidism),
— diabetes mellitus,
— pregnancy,
— use of certain medications, alcohol, narcotics.
In a large number of patients, however, no clear cause can be found, in which case the disorder is called **"idiopathic" ("functional" or "non-ulcer") dyspepsia**.

In diagnosing a patient with dyspeptic symptoms, the doctor must make full use of his or her knowledge, experience, and intuition. He or she must be on the alert for signs of certain disorders.

If there is no evidence of a serious underlying disorder, one should first attempt to identify:
— symptoms such as observed in ulcer (especially **"ulcer-like"** pain)
— symptoms such as are found in gastro-oesophageal reflux (**"reflux-like"** heartburn and similar complaints
— symptoms such as occur in disordered gastric emptying (**"dysmotility-like"** epigastric fullness, nausea).
A drug is chosen by way of institution of a trial treatment on the basis of the type of symptoms: for ulcer-like symptoms an H_2-blocker, for reflux-like complaints a prokinetic, H_2-blocker or mucosa protectant, and for dysmotility-like symptoms a prokinetic. It should be remembered that disordered gastric emptying is the most frequent symptom of dyspepsia and that a disordered gastric emptying can cause reflux and ulcer-like symptoms. In some patients reflux symptoms dominate the picture to such an extent that these should be investigated first (Figure 108, p. 228). If a treatment for reflux is inadequate, gastric function should be further examined (according to Figure 109, p. 230). Only in special cases (p. 108) should gastric function be investigated by means, amongst other methods, of a gastric emptying study, manometry or EGG.
The motility of the oesophagus and LOS can be inhibited by **drugs** (cf. Table 3, p. 71). In particular muscarinic blockers (or drugs with an anticholinergic component) exert this type of effect. Pharmacological actions must be kept in mind during the history taking. If one

wishes to stimulate gastric motility with a prokinetic that releases acetylcholine, one must ensure that the patient is not using drugs with an antimuscarinic (side-)effect at the same time. The latter type of drug would neutralize the action of the prokinetic.

Gastritis and duodenitis are frequently detected by means of endoscopy. In working out a strategy it is important to distinguish the erosive from the non-erosive forms.

◆ Erosive gastritis and duodenitis can be accompanied by ulcer-like pain. Patients with these disorders generally respond well to H_2-blockers.
◆ Chronic non-erosive gastritis (and duodenitis) are often found in symptom-free persons (Intermezzo 29). Gastritis (or duodenitis) by itself, therefore, does not constitute a reason for treatment.

Non-erosive gastritis and duodenitis are much more prevalent than the erosive forms.

Intermezzo 29
***Helicobacter pylori*: A contributory factor?**

For some time much attention has been focused on *Helicobacter pylori** This bacterium was suspected of provoking gastritis, ulcer and dyspeptic symptoms. If that were correct, an efficacious, causal treatment of dyspeptic symptoms would be possible. In this connection, hopes were vested in bismuth subcitrate, a mucosa protectant with some antibacterial activity. It is now believed that *Helicobacter pylori* contributes little to dyspeptic symptoms. And if it does contribute to them, there are more effective therapies than bactericides. This conclusion is based on the following observations:
◆ It is generally held that *Helicobacter pylori* causes aspecific gastritis. But a large portion of the population has the form of gastritis associated with *Helicobacter pylori* without any symptoms.
◆ Bismuth subcitrate is not a very effective antibacterial against *Helicobacter pylori;* in monotherapy with bismuth subcitrate the bacteria is eliminated in only 20–25% of the patients.
◆ It is possible that *Helicobacter pylori* plays a role in the pathogenesis of erosive gastritis and bulbitis and gastric and duodenal ulcer, but these disorders are effectively treated with H_2-blockers. Only in exceptional cases is the total elimination of *Helicobacter pylori* indicated. Reference is made here uniquely to patients with very frequently recurring duodenal ulcer, in which case a combination of antibiotics (e.g. metronidazole, bismuth subcitrate and amoxicillin) is prescribed.

---

* This bacterium was formerly called *Campylobacter pylori.*

Delayed gastric emptying is found in the following disorders and situations:

Acute:
— abdominal pain, trauma, inflammations
— postoperative status (ileus)
— infections, gastroenteritis
— metabolic disorders (acidosis, hypokalaemia, hyper- or hypocalcaemia, hyperglycaemia, hepatic coma, uraemia
— immobilization

Chronic:
— gastric ulcer
— diabetes mellitus (diabetic visceral neuropathy)
— atrophic gastritis
— vagotomy (sometimes unintentional when fundoplication is performed to prevent reflux)
— partial gastrectomy with a Roux-en-Y reconstruction
— intracerebral disorders
— systemic sclerosis
— dermatomyositis
— familial visceral myopathy
— muscle disease (e.g. myotonic dystrophy)
— infiltrative disease (carcinoma, amyloidosis)
— hypothyroidism
— achlorhydria
— pseudo-obstruction (idiopathic or secondary)
— idiopathic gastric dysrhythmia (tachygastria)
— idiopathic gastroduodenal dyssynchronia
— anorexia nervosa
— psychogenic vomiting

Acute or chronic:
— mechanical obstruction
— drugs: morphinomimetic agents, anticholinergic agents, L-dopa, psychotropic agents, aluminium hydroxide
— pregnancy
— tabes dorsalis

Table 9: Delayed gastric emptying.

Diarrhoea

In diagnosing a patient with diarrhoea, the doctor must rely to a large extent on his or her experience and intuition. Diarrhoea can be a symptom of a large number of different disorders.

First, one should attempt to determine if **infections** caused by viruses, bacteria or parasites are a contributory factor (Figure 112, p. 236). It is also important to ascertain whether the patient uses an excessive quantity of laxatives.

In a number of patients, diarrhoea is cause by food. In this connection a distinction is made between **food allergy** and **food intolerance.** Numerous foods can provoke food allergy. With intolerance, one should be on the lookout for lactose, gluten, spicy food and food additives.

A number of diseases are attended by (secondary) dysmotility of the large intestine, which can give rise to diarrhoea. We are thinking here of **inflammatory bowel disease** (IBD, an umbrella term for ulcerative colitis and Crohn's disease).

Accelerated gastric emptying often develops in the following situations:

— after a highly selective vagotomy (liquids)
— truncal vagotomy with or without pyloroplasty (liquids)
— partial gastrectomy (B-I or B-II)
— hyperthyroidism
— exocrine pancreatic insufficiency
— Zollinger-Ellison syndrome
— duodenal ulcer disease

Table 10: Accelerated gastric emptying.

Pain in the lower abdomen

Pain in the lower abdomen can result from motility disorders of the small or large intestine but also from a number of organic disturbances (Figure 110, p. 232). The most likely pathologies are as follows:
— colon carcinoma,
— obstruction of the small intestine (e.g. in Crohn's disease),
— appendicitis,
— disorders of the urinary bladder, uterus, adnexa uteri.

Also, if the patient feels pain mainly in the lower abdomen, the cause may well be located in the upper abdomen (e.g. in peptic ulcer).

The motility of the small and large intestines can be inhibited by **drugs** (cf. Table 3, p. 71), which can bring about an ileus-like picture. Muscarinic blockers (or drugs with an anticholinergic component) act in this fashion. This pharmacological action must be kept in mind while taking the history.

If a **gastric, duodenal or colonic disorder** is suspected, an endoscopy or radiographic examination of these organs should be performed.

If a **total obstruction of the small or large intestine** is suspected, a plain film of the abdomen (without contrast medium) should be taken (p. 283). In a supine patient with ileus, dilation of the loops of the small and/or large intestine is observed and in a standing patient there are air fluid levels in the intestinal loops. In (pseudo)obstruction of the small or large intestine, identical images are observed; it is generally impossible to distinguish between an organic and a pseudo-obstruction on the basis of an X-ray. If there is solid evidence of an obstruction ileus, an immediate laparotomy is indicated. The diagnosis is made with the abdomen open.

If a **motility disorder of the small or large intestine** is suspected, a radiographic examination yields the most important information. A plain film of the abdomen can also be useful in revealing an accumulation of faecal material in the large intestine. Sometimes it is desirable to do supplementary barium or double-contrast radiography. Transit disorders of the small intestine can be quantified scintigraphically or by means of the breath hydrogen test. To study large intestinal transit one can have the patient swallow beads or rings, which can be followed radiographically or scintigraphically (Figure 126, p. 285). The movements of the colon are more difficult to study. Colonic spasms are sometimes disclosed on X-rays or endoscopically (Figure 85, p. 159). Manometry of the colon is in principle suitable for studying the movements of the colon but it is still limited to research use.

Unexplained pain in the lower abdomen accompanied by constipation, diarrhoea or alternating constipation and diarrhoea is generally diagnosed as **IBS** (cf. p. 158).

Constipation

In diagnosing patients with constipation a number of well-defined critical choices must be made (Figure 111, p. 234). In a theoretical scheme, the questions always lead to unequivocal decisions but in reality the procedure is much more complex.

"Suspect" or (probably) "not suspect"?

In a number of patients with constipation there are reasons to suspect an obstruction due to tumour, diverticulitis, Crohn's disease or an anatomical abnormality of the anorectal region. Radiographic examination, colonoscopy and sigmoidoscopy are suitable techniques for disclosing or excluding these disorders.

Trial treatment or further examination?

Generally constipation is a non-malignant symptom. The right diet and, when appropriate, the use of laxatives is often sufficient to keep the symptoms under control. In addition, constipation can occur as the side-effect of a drug. Muscarinic blockers (or drugs with anticholinergic side-effects) and opiates* can contribute to this effect.

Colonic or anorectal disorder?

With constipation it is important to determine the primary site of the disturbance of passage of the faeces: in the colon or in the anorectal region. The questions asked while taking the history should be chosen to make this distinction.

- If the patient regularly experiences the defaecation urge, but cannot expel the faeces, there is probably an anorectal disorder.
- If the patient rarely experiences a defaecation urge (three times per week or less), generally it is the colonic passage that is impaired. In that case the faeces reach the anorectal junction less frequently.
- There is, however, a small group of patients that seldom or never experience the defaecation urge but nonetheless have an anorectal disorder. Their problem is a loss of anorectal sensitivity: the faeces arrive in the anorectal region but the patient can't perceive the event.

Disordered colonic transit?

- Constipation can occur secondarily to other disorders, like systemic sclerosis, diabetes mellitus, hypothyroidism, myotonic dystrophy and neuropathology.
- Severe constipation can be life-threatening. In this connection one need merely call to mind inert colon, CIIP and Ogilvie's syndrome.

Disordered anorectal transit?

In patients with disturbed anorectal passage one should attempt to establish the primary cause of the constipation: a **dysmotility** (anismus, Hirschsprung's disease, impaired sensitivity) or an **anatomical abnormality.** For a reliable diagnosis of the most frequent motility disorders of the rectum and pelvic floor, manometry, EMG, defaecography or a biopsy are necessary. If an anatomical abnormality of the anorectal region is found, it should be remembered that this does not always cause constipation. Sometimes the anatomical abnormality is the result of constipation (hard straining) and sometimes it is merely an attendant phenomenon.

---

* An overdose of antidiarrhoeals can also provoke constipation.

Incontinence

If a patient presents with incontinence, attention should also be focused on the most obvious causes of this disorder (Figure 113, p. 238): dementia, CVA or trauma (whether or not as a result of difficult labour). When the incontinence is accompanied by constipation, one should first consider the constipation; if this can be reduced, the incontinence will also often subside. In the ensuing examinations, **anatomical abnormalities** should be focused on (e.g. external prolapse). Next, one should try to differentiate between the following (Table 11):
— myogenic incontinence
— neurogenic incontinence
— idiopathic (unexplained) incontinence.

Sphincter impairment can often be found at the physical examination. Anal digital examination can provide some information about sphincter tone, squeeze pressure, possible asymmetry of the sphincter, puborectal muscle tone (a global impression) and the presence of a palpable occult prolapse. A diminished or asymmetric anal sphincter tone can indicate muscle damage or defective innervation. Anal endosonography is an excellent means of detecting damage to the anal sphincters. Anatomical abnormalities in the anorectal region can also be identified by means of sigmoidoscopy. Sometimes there is solid evidence of neurogenic incontinence (e.g. CVA, dementia, multiple sclerosis or diabetes mellitus). It is much more difficult to identify unequivocally lesions of the pudential nerve. (Only in certain centres

study method	myogenic	neurogenic
direct observation or anal endosonography	muscle damage	no muscle damage
manometry	asymmetric pressure profile	pressure profile usually symmetrical
EMG	low amplitude (often locally lower)	— low activity — abnormal motor unit potentials — denervation potentials — reinnervation potentials — diminished conduction velocity of the pudendal nerve

Table 11: Differentiation of myogenic from neurogenic incontinence.

is this possible.) To do this an EMG of
the individual muscle fibres is
performed and the conduction velocity
of the pudendal nerve is measured. In
many patients with so-called idiopathic
incontinence, pudendal impairment can
be disclosed by a special study. It is then
seen that these patients have
neurogenic incontinence.

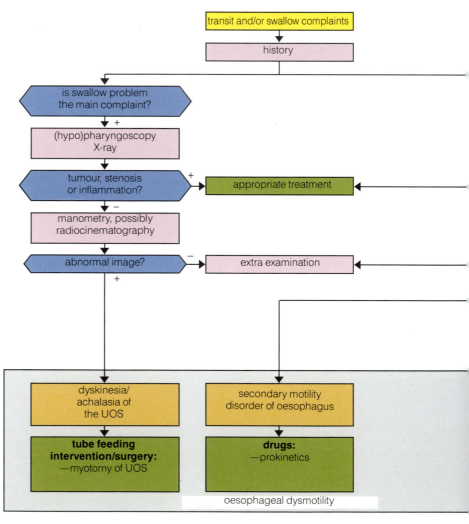

Figure 107: Flow chart for diagnosing patients presenting with mainly swallow and oesophageal transit symptoms.

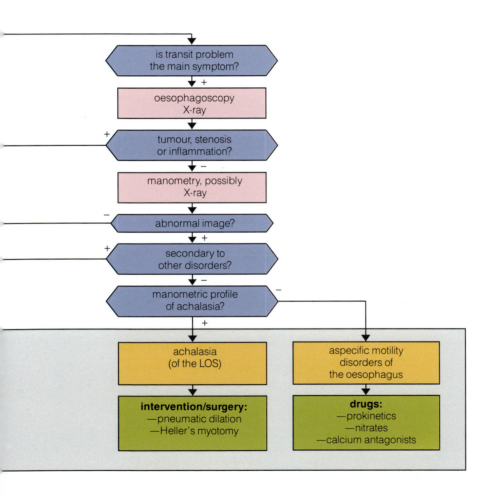

is transit problem
the main symptom?

+

oesophagoscopy
X-ray

+ tumour, stenosis
or inflammation?

−

manometry, possibly
X-ray

− abnormal image?

+

+ secondary to
other disorders?

−

manometric profile
of achalasia? −

+

achalasia
(of the LOS)

aspecific motility
disorders of
the oesophagus

intervention/surgery:
—pneumatic dilation
—Heller's myotomy

drugs:
—prokinetics
—nitrates
—calcium antagonists

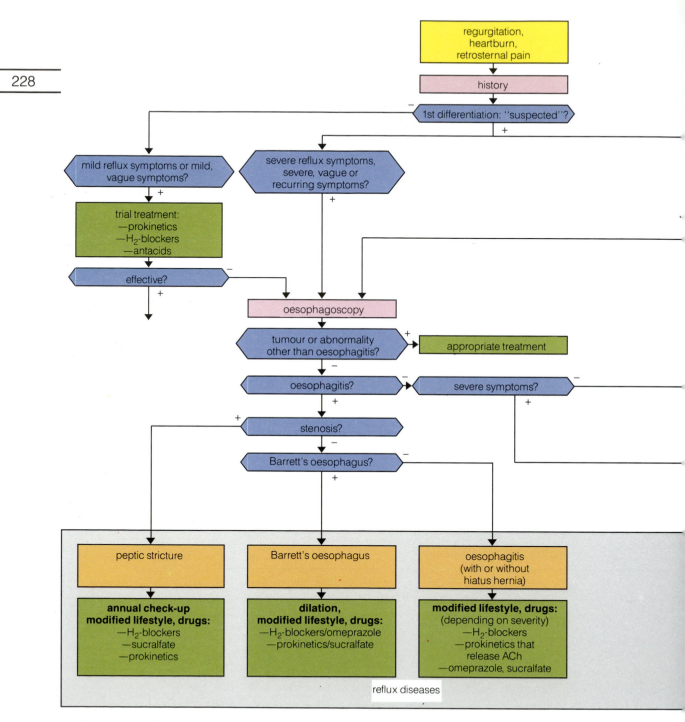

Figure 108: Flow chart for diagnosing patients presenting with symptoms mainly related to gastro-oesophageal reflux: regurgitation, heartburn, and retrosternal pain.

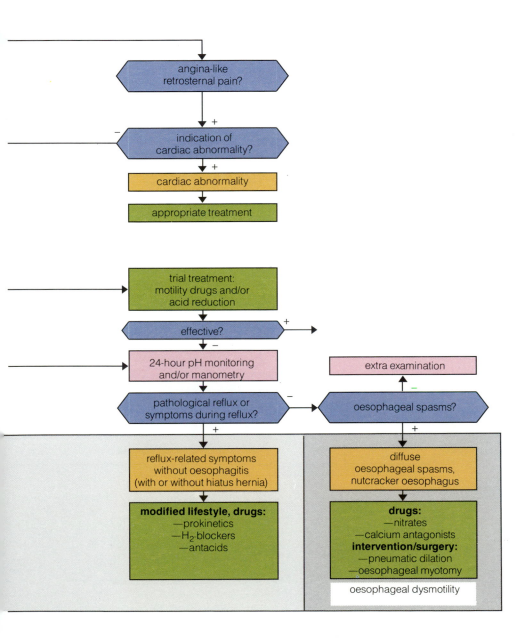

angina-like
retrosternal pain?

− indication of
cardiac abnormality? +

+

cardiac abnormality

appropriate treatment

trial treatment:
motility drugs and/or
acid reduction

effective? +

−

24-hour pH monitoring
and/or manometry

extra examination

pathological reflux or
symptoms during reflux? − oesophageal spasms? −

+ +

reflux-related symptoms
without oesophagitis
(with or without hiatus hernia)

diffuse
oesophageal spasms,
nutcracker oesophagus

modified lifestyle, drugs:
—prokinetics
—H$_2$-blockers
—antacids

drugs:
—nitrates
—calcium antagonists
intervention/surgery:
—pneumatic dilation
—oesophageal myotomy

oesophageal dysmotility

D I A G N O S I S

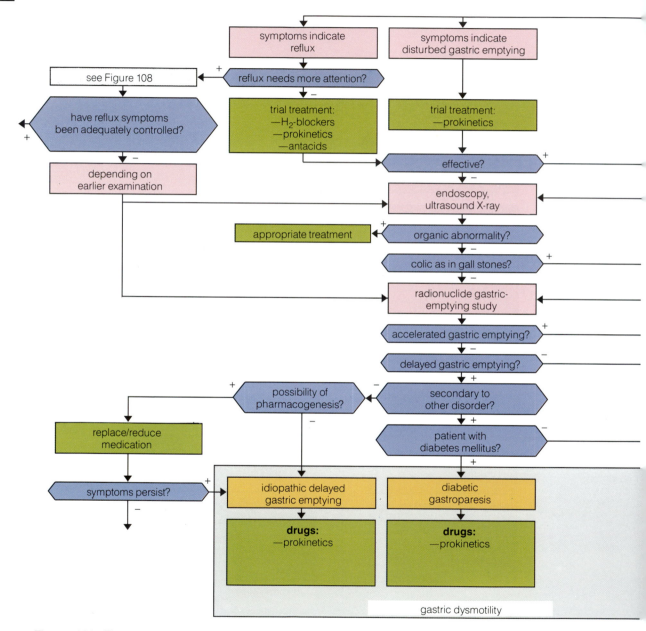

Figure 109: Flow chart for diagnosing patients presenting with mainly dyspeptic symptoms.

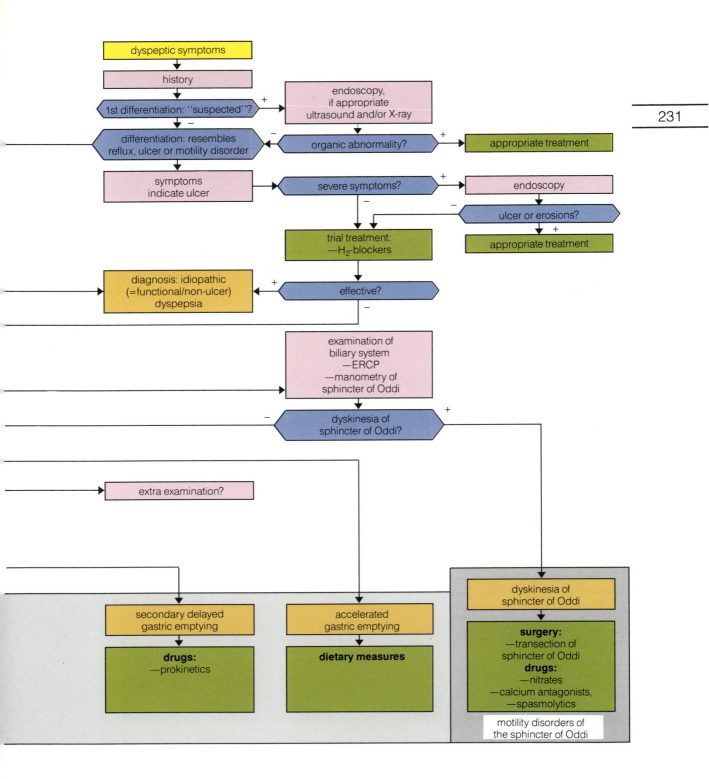

dyspeptic symptoms

history

1st differentiation: "suspected"? → + → endoscopy, if appropriate ultrasound and/or X-ray

− differentiation: resembles reflux, ulcer or motility disorder ← − organic abnormality? → + → appropriate treatment

symptoms indicate ulcer → severe symptoms? → + → endoscopy

− ulcer or erosions? → + → appropriate treatment

trial treatment: —H₂-blockers

diagnosis: idiopathic (=functional/non-ulcer) dyspepsia ← + effective? −

examination of biliary system —ERCP —manometry of sphincter of Oddi

− dyskinesia of sphincter of Oddi? +

extra examination?

secondary delayed gastric emptying
drugs: —prokinetics

accelerated gastric emptying
dietary measures

dyskinesia of sphincter of Oddi
surgery: —transection of sphincter of Oddi drugs: —nitrates —calcium antagonists, —spasmolytics

motility disorders of the sphincter of Oddi

DIAGNOSIS

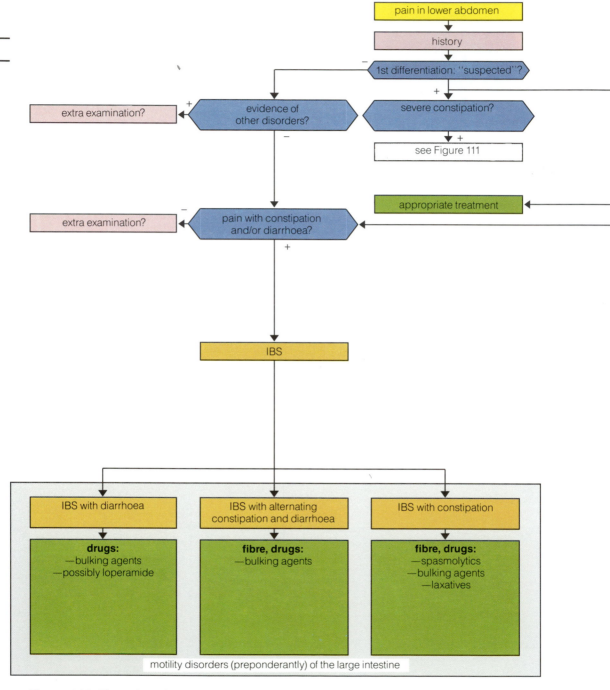

Figure 110: Flow chart for diagnosing patients with pain in the lower abdomen as the main presenting symptom.

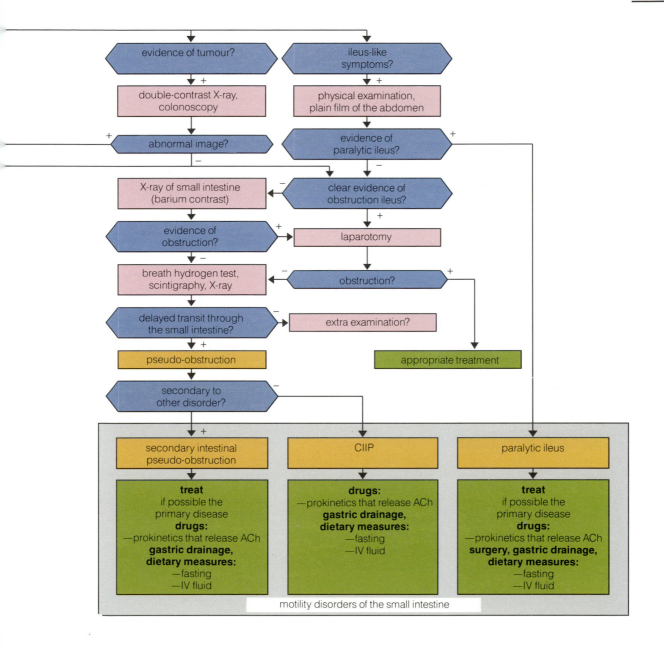

evidence of tumour?

+

double-contrast X-ray, colonoscopy

ileus-like symptoms?

+

physical examination, plain film of the abdomen

+

abnormal image?

evidence of paralytic ileus?

+

−

−

X-ray of small intestine (barium contrast)

clear evidence of obstruction ileus?

−

+

evidence of obstruction?

+

laparotomy

−

breath hydrogen test, scintigraphy, X-ray

obstruction?

−

+

delayed transit through the small intestine?

−

extra examination?

+

pseudo-obstruction

appropriate treatment

secondary to other disorder?

−

+

secondary intestinal pseudo-obstruction

CIIP

paralytic ileus

treat
if possible the
primary disease
drugs:
—prokinetics that release ACh
**gastric drainage,
dietary measures:**
—fasting
—IV fluid

drugs:
—prokinetics that release ACh
**gastric drainage,
dietary measures:**
—fasting
—IV fluid

treat
if possible the
primary disease
drugs:
—prokinetics that release ACh
**surgery, gastric drainage,
dietary measures:**
—fasting
—IV fluid

motility disorders of the small intestine

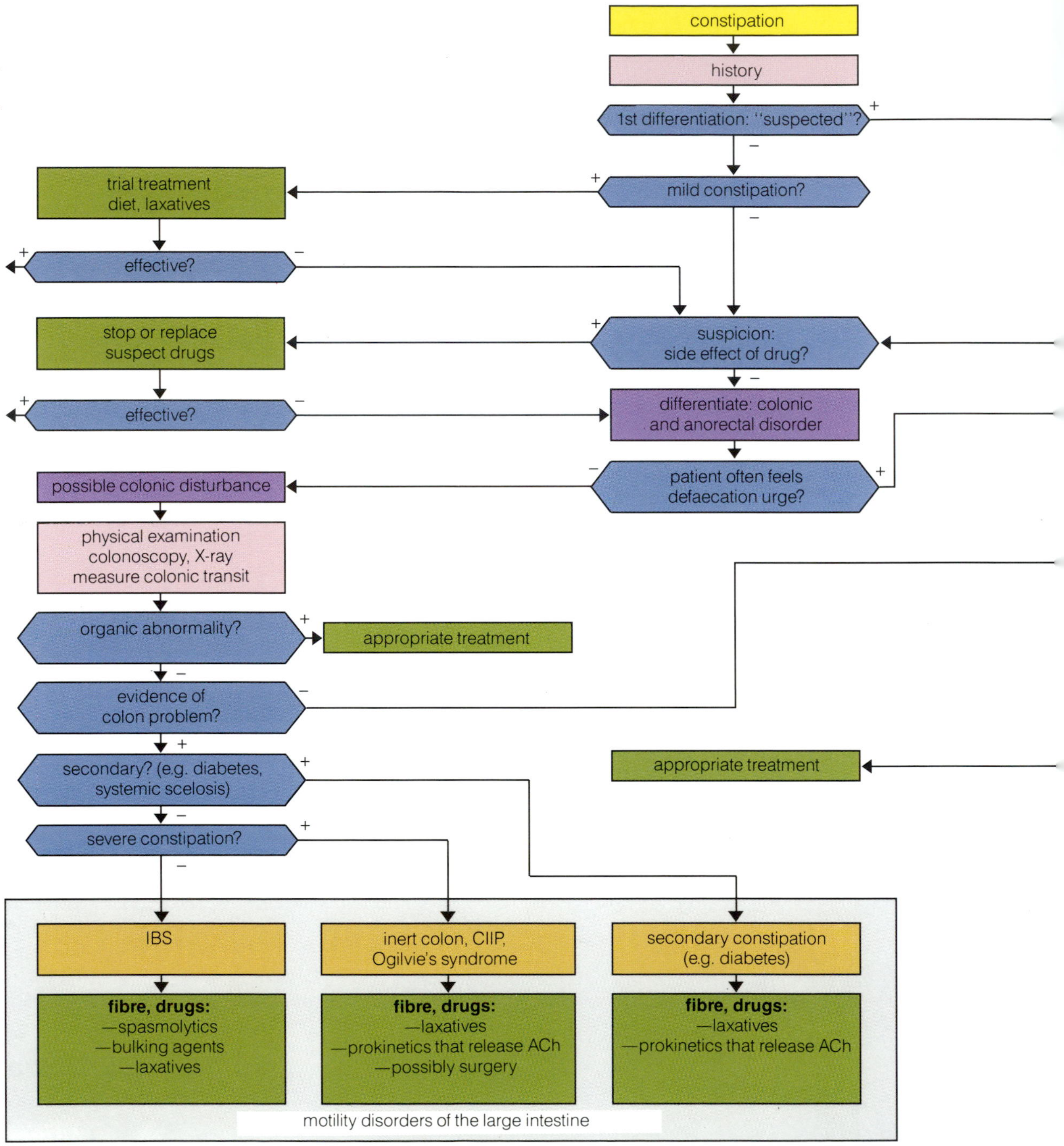

Figure 111: Flow chart for diagnosing patients presenting with constipation as the main symptom.

The flow chart contains the following elements:

- constipation
- history
- 1st differentiation: "suspected"? (+ / −)
- mild constipation? (+ / −)
  - + → trial treatment diet, laxatives
    - effective? (+ / −)
- suspicion: side effect of drug? (+ / −)
  - + → stop or replace suspect drugs
    - effective? (+ / −)
- differentiate: colonic and anorectal disorder
- patient often feels defaecation urge? (+ / −)
  - − → possible colonic disturbance
    - physical examination colonoscopy, X-ray measure colonic transit
    - organic abnormality? (+ / −)
      - + → appropriate treatment
    - evidence of colon problem? (+ / −)
    - secondary? (e.g. diabetes, systemic sclerosis) (+ / −)
    - severe constipation? (+ / −)
- appropriate treatment

motility disorders of the large intestine:

- IBS
  - fibre, drugs:
    —spasmolytics
    —bulking agents
    —laxatives
- inert colon, CIIP, Ogilvie's syndrome
  - fibre, drugs:
    —laxatives
    —prokinetics that release ACh
    —possibly surgery
- secondary constipation (e.g. diabetes)
  - fibre, drugs:
    —laxatives
    —prokinetics that release ACh

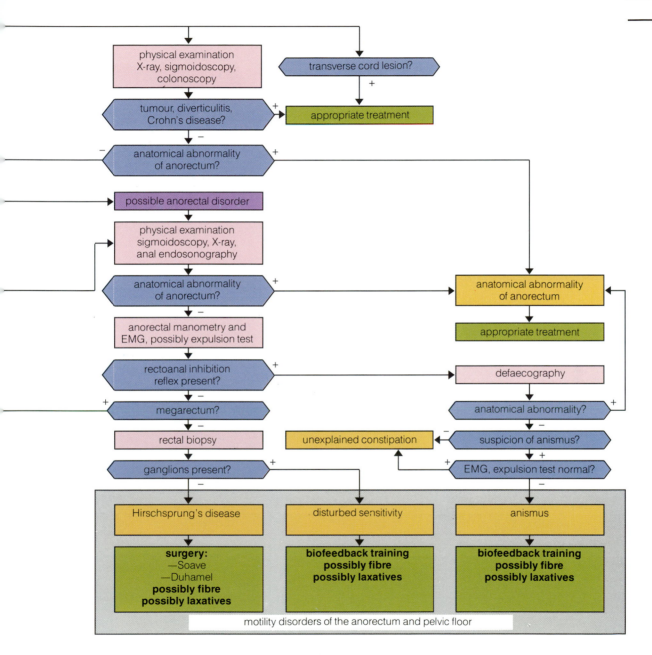

physical examination
X-ray, sigmoidoscopy,
colonoscopy

transverse cord lesion?

+

tumour, diverticulitis,
Crohn's disease?

+

appropriate treatment

−

anatomical abnormality
of anorectum?

+

possible anorectal disorder

physical examination
sigmoidoscopy, X-ray,
anal endosonography

anatomical abnormality
of anorectum?

+

anatomical abnormality
of anorectum

−

appropriate treatment

anorectal manometry and
EMG, possibly expulsion test

−

rectoanal inhibition
reflex present?

+

defaecography

−

megarectum?

+

anatomical abnormality?

+

−

rectal biopsy

unexplained constipation

−

suspicion of anismus?

ganglions present?

+

+

EMG, expulsion test normal?

−

−

Hirschsprung's disease

disturbed sensitivity

anismus

surgery:
—Soave
—Duhamel
**possibly fibre
possibly laxatives**

**biofeedback training
possibly fibre
possibly laxatives**

**biofeedback training
possibly fibre
possibly laxatives**

motility disorders of the anorectum and pelvic floor

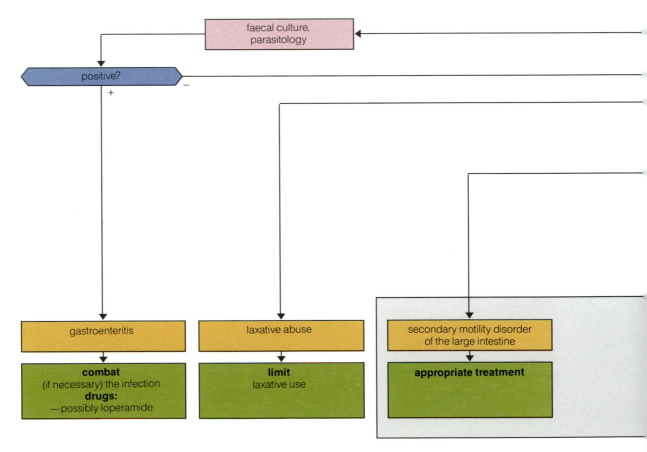

Figure 112: Flow chart for diagnosing patients presenting with diarrhoea as the main complaint.

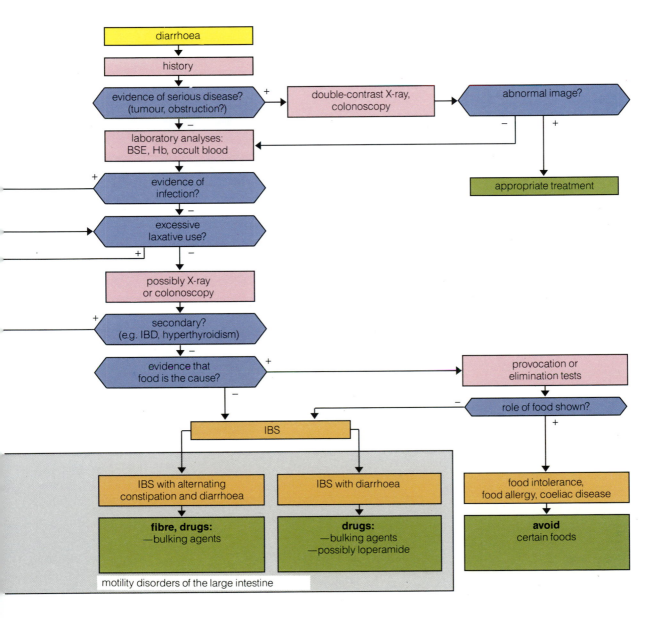

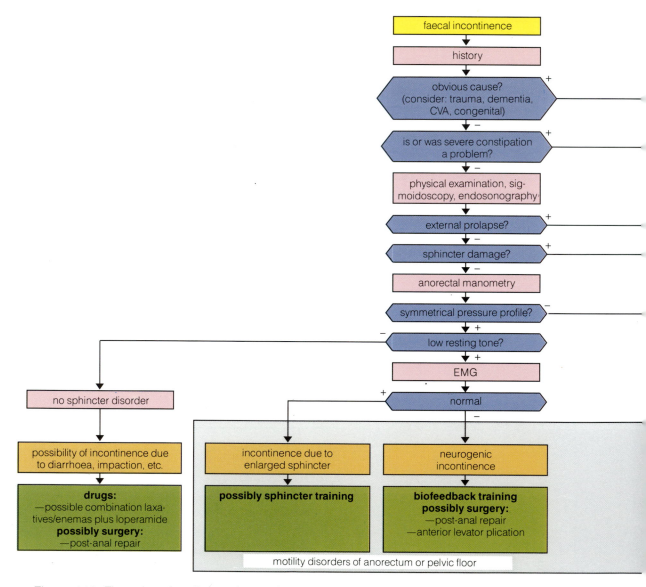

Figure 113: Flow chart for diagnosing patients presenting with faecal incontinence as the main symptom.

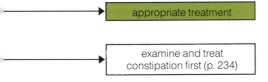

appropriate treatment

examine and treat
constipation first (p. 234)

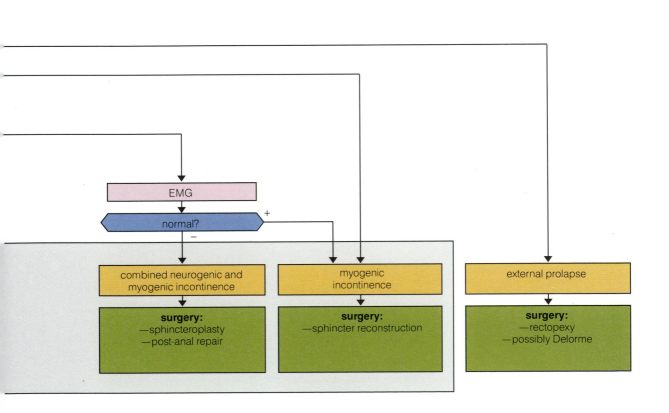

EMG

normal?

+

−

combined neurogenic and
myogenic incontinence

myogenic
incontinence

external prolapse

surgery:
—sphincteroplasty
—post-anal repair

surgery:
—sphincter reconstruction

surgery:
—rectopexy
—possibly Delorme

Chapter 13

Diseases associated with generalized motility disorders of the gastrointestinal tract

In certain diseases, (secondary) motility disorders occur in large parts of the gastrointestinal tract. It is important to identify these since a number of patients respond favourably to drug therapy.

Introduction

Earlier in this book mention was made of frequently occurring diseases attended by (secondary) generalized motility disorders. Here we shall elaborate on these since it is important for the attending physician to be able to identify them. It is self-evident that fruitless diagnoses and surgery can be avoided as a result of early detection. Moreover, the motility disorders of these patients can often be treated with drugs. In this way at least their gastrointestinal problems can be relieved.

Chronic idiopathic intestinal pseudo-obstruction (CIIP)

For decades it has been known that some patients present the clinical picture of chronic obstruction of the small intestine without an obstruction being present. Some of these patients have another disease (i.e. diabetes mellitus, systemic sclerosis, muscular dystrophy) that is sometimes accompanied by motility disorders of the gastrointestinal tract. In addition, intestinal transit can be impeded by drugs, especially by muscarinic blockers (or drugs that have antimuscarinic, "anticholinergic" side-effects) and opiates.

The recognition of CIIP
But there is another group of patients for whom the clinical picture of obstruction could not be explained and was serious enough to warrant surgery. During the operation, however, no obstruction or lesion was found and after the operation the symptoms persisted or recurred. A second operation was performed in search of adhesions from the first, and so on. Patients often showed up with a "battlefield abdomen", displaying the scars of a hopeless search for an obstruction. Finally, the name "chronic idiopathic intestinal pseudo-obstruction" (CIIP) was accepted for this disorder. CIIP was recognized and accepted as a disorder only after obstruction was excluded as a cause in enough patients, each of whom first underwent several operations. Since that time we have learned much about this pathology.

CIIP is often familial

It has been discovered that intestinal pseudo-obstruction tends to run in certain families. There is strong evidence of a hereditary component of variable expression. The mechanism of transmission is not yet understood. It is even suspected that the term CIIP covers several disorders with different transmission mechanisms. The symptoms are manifested mostly in young adults. The disorder was and is fatal. Once it was recognized that CIIP was a familial disorder, it was realized that not only the patient but also his or her relatives needed to be examined. This circumstance made further-reaching investigation possible.

CIIP affects the entire gastrointestinal tract

When it is recognized that a patient has CIIP, examination of relatives often reveals various disorders spread over the entire gastrointestinal tract and also, for example, the urinary bladder and the musculus sphincter pupillae. (Some patients have large pupils.) Various diagnoses can be found in the families (Table 12). A number of members of a CIIP patient's family do not have any symptoms at all, but when they are examined radiographically, abnormalities are disclosed, like dilated stomach, megaduodenum, megacolon and megacystis.

CIIP is often induced by myopathy or neuropathy

Two groups of CIIP patients can be identified by means of a histological examination.

◆ Patients with **myopathy**. Usually there is progressive degeneration of the smooth muscle and fibrosis. Histological examination reveals that the smooth muscle of parts of the gastrointestinal tract or the urinary bladder and urinary tracts also degenerate.

◆ Patients with **neuropathy**. In CIIP with neuropathy there are generally severe symptoms from birth, but sometimes as well later in life. The neurons of the myenteric plexus are present in rudimentary form or they are degenerate. In the worst cases, there are no neurons. Food intake via the mouth is impossible and the prognosis is poor (some babies survive a few months due to intravenous feeding). In other cases the neuropathy is limited to the large intestine, as a result of which there is constipation from birth. The patients respond quite well to colonic resection.

Myopathy and neuropathy can also be differentiated by means of manometry (p. 140).

location	previous diagnosis
oesophagus	achalasia
stomach	pyloric stenosis
duodenum	superior mesenteric artery syndrome
small intestine	adhesions, Crohn's disease, coeliac disease refractory to gluten elimination
large intestine and rectum	irritable bowel syndrome, Hirschsprung's disease
urinary bladder	neurogenic bladder
general	anorexia nervosa

Table 12: Examples of incorrect first diagnoses in familial CIIP. (Modified, from Christensen and Anuras, 1983.)

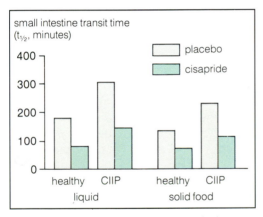

Figure 114: Small intestine transit time for liquid and solid food is longer in CIIP. Cisapride accelerates this transit. (Reproduced with permission, from Camilleri et al., 1986.)

Patients with CIIP respond quite favourably to prokinetics

It is important for the patient that CIIP should be correctly diagnosed since it can be a fatal disease, and whether it is or not, it is always accompanied by severe symptoms. Formerly the treatment consisted of stimulating intestinal motility with cholinesterase antagonists, but these drugs have many side-effects. A number of patients respond well to prokinetics that liberate acetylcholine. Cisapride accelerates gastric emptying and transit through the small intestine in patients with CIIP (Figure 114). Their symptoms are substantially reduced. In CIIP good results can be expected from cisapride provided that enough neurons and smooth muscle cells are still viable.

Diabetes mellitus

Gastrointestinal symptoms occur frequently in diabetes but are often overlooked because other problems appear to be more serious. However, although a diabetes patient can be prescribed a detailed diet, if gastrointestinal motility is disordered, the food uptake is abnormal. Even an elaborate diet can then give little relief. Gastrointestinal symptoms are frequent in both insulin-dependent (type I) and insulin-independent (type II) diabetes mellitus.

Complications in diabetes mellitus
In diabetes a broad range of complications occur, which can give rise to different symptoms. It is often a burdensome task to sort out the factors to which certain symptoms should be primarily attributed. A well-known complication of diabetes is progressive neuropathy, a relentlessly invasive degeneration of the peripheral and enteric nerve cells. In diabetes the glucose balance (by definition) and the electrolyte balance are dysregulated. This situation can lead to a wide range of complications. In addition, there are hormonal abnormalities and the patients are more liable to bacterial and fungal infections.

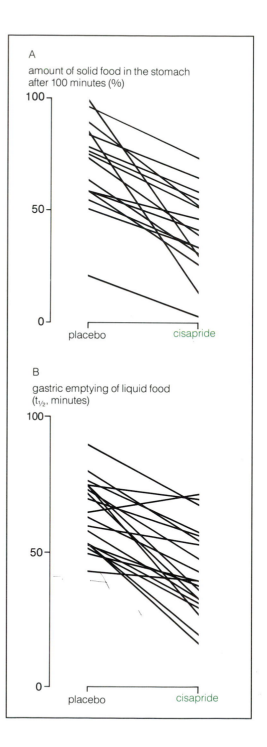

Figure 115: Cisapride accelerates gastric emptying of liquids and solids in diabetes mellitus. (Reproduced with permission, from Horowitz et al., 1987b.)

Gastrointestinal symptoms in diabetes mellitus

Closer examination reveals that up to 75% of patients with diabetes also have gastrointestinal symptoms. Diabetic gastroparesis is fairly familiar, but higher and lower in the digestive tract diminished motility has been discovered. The main symptom is constipation but dysphagia, reflux symptoms, dyspepsia and abdominal pain are also observed. Diabetes patients have delayed gastric emptying and a delayed intestinal transit. A special problem in diabetes is that often phase III of the MMC is absent. And this is precisely the phase in which indigestible particles leave the stomach. In these patients large indigestible particles remain in the stomach for an inordinately long time. It is generally believed that these motility disorders are caused by autonomic or enteric neuropathy, but hyperglycaemia, infections and hormonal abnormalities can also cause them.

Prokinetics in patients with diabetes mellitus

Prokinetics promote the motility of the digestive tract in diabetics. Gastric emptying in these patients is initially accelerated by domperidone and metoclopramide but the effect often wears off after a short treatment (1 month). In contrast, cisapride accelerates gastric emptying more potently and is longer acting in a larger portion of diabetes mellitus patients (Figure 115). Prokinetics are also capable of stimulating the digestion of indigestible particles. In this respect cisapride is more effective than metoclopramide (Figure 116).

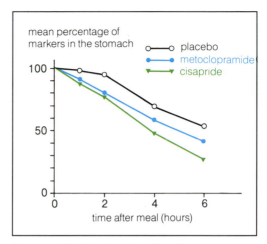

Figure 116: Prokinetics that liberate acetylcholine accelerate gastric emptying of indigestible particles in diabetes mellitus patients (data recorded by scintigraphy). Both drugs were intravenously administered (metoclopramide 10 mg, cisapride 5 mg). Cisapride is more effective. (Reproduced with permission, from Feldman and Smith, 1987.)

Systemic sclerosis

Systemic sclerosis is a severe form of connective tissue degeneration. The connective tissue in various tissues and organs can be affected. In some patients only one or two organs are affected and in some several. Also, abnormalities are found of the skin (hardening mainly of the hands and face), bones, gastrointestinal tract, liver, kidneys, lungs, heart and muscles. Because hardening of the skin is the most striking characteristic, this disease is also called "scleroderma"*. Often Raynaud's phenomenon is the first sign of the disorder. If calcinosis (calcium salt deposition in soft tissue), Raynaud's phenomenon, "oesophageal involvement", sclerodactyly and telangiectasias are present, the condition is referred to as the "Crest syndrome". Systemic sclerosis is a rare disease: the incidence is two to seven patients per year per million persons. There are no reliable data on its cause.

The gastrointestinal tract in systemic sclerosis

In systemic sclerosis abnormalities can be observed over the entire gastrointestinal tract.

◆ **The oesophagus**. In most patients with systemic sclerosis the oesophagus is affected. Reflux symptoms are most frequent whilst dysphagia also occurs. Examination often discloses a dilated, atonic oesophagus; peristaltic contractions are disordered or even absent.

◆ **The stomach**. In most patients with systemic sclerosis the stomach is more or less spared. Occasionally the stomach is distended and lacks peristaltic contractions.

◆ The **small intestine**. In systemic sclerosis the small intestine often produces too few peristaltic contractions. Transit through it is therefore substantially delayed and symptoms manifest themselves that are characteristic of obstruction. Bacterial overgrowth is often observed. Paralytic ileus in systemic sclerosis is life-threatening.

◆ The **large intestine**. In many patients with systemic sclerosis the movements of the large intestine are also disordered, resulting in constipation and diarrhoea.

*Systemic sclerosis must be clearly differentiated from circumscript scleroderma, which manifests itself as a circumscribed skin abnormality on the trunk.

Prokinetics in systemic sclerosis

It is possible in patients with systemic sclerosis to stimulate gastrointestinal motility. Cisapride stimulates oesophageal motility and promotes oesophageal clearance. It also raises the LOS pressure. In addition, cisapride stimulates the gastric motility of patients with systemic sclerosis and gastric emptying of liquids is therefore accelerated (Figure 117). It follows that this drug reduces reflux and dyspeptic symptoms in systemic sclerosis patients.

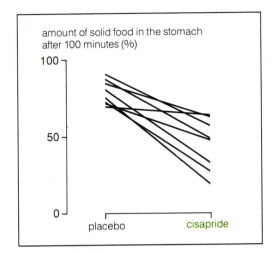

Figure 117: Cisapride accelerates gastric emptying of solid food in patients with systemic sclerosis. (Reproduced with permission, from Horowitz et al., 1987c.)

Muscular dystrophy

Motility disorders of the gastrointestinal tract can occur in muscular dystrophy. Gastrointestinal complications have been further examined in two forms. Duchenne type muscular dystrophy (dystrophia musculorum) and myotonic dystrophy.

Duchenne type muscular dystrophy

Duchenne type muscular dystrophy (often called simply "muscular dystrophy") is a dramatically developing hereditary disease. It is recessively transmitted and the gene is located on the x-chromosome. It is therefore found almost exclusively in boys. About 30 in 100,000 boys born alive suffer from it. Its victims usually die from it before age 20 years.

Gastrointestinal complications from Duchenne's disease

In patients with Duchenne's disease not only the striated muscle but also the smooth muscle is affected. Frequently gastrointestinal complications develop. The symptoms are vomiting, epigastric pain, abdominal pain and diarrhoea. A distended stomach and signs of intestinal obstruction (pseudo-obstruction) are observed. Gastric emptying is delayed. As far as we know it has not been attempted to stimulate the gastrointestinal motility in these patients with prokinetics that liberate acetylcholine, although this is a rational strategy.

Myotonic dystrophy

Myotonic dystrophy (Curschmann-Steinert syndrome) is typically associated with atrophy of the striated muscles of, amongst other regions, the face, neck, hands and lower legs. At the same time there is myotony of the striated muscles, i.e. after contraction the muscles contract very slowly. The diagnosis is made on the basis of the striking EMG. The disease is transmitted by a dominant gene located on chromosome 19. Generally the signs and symptoms of it manifest themselves in puberty or in young adults, but also in 20% of newborns. It is a relatively benign form of muscular dystrophy. It is the most frequent form of muscular dystrophy in adults. Its incidence is 13 per 100,000 living newborns and its prevalence 2–6 inhabitants per 100,000.

The gastrointestinal tract in myotonic dystrophy

In myotonic dystrophy not only striated muscle but also smooth muscle is affected. In 80% of patients with myotonic dystrophy, gastrointestinal symptoms are found: dysphagia, dyspepsia, abdominal cramps, constipation and diarrhoea. Oesophageal and gastric emptying are delayed and the motility of the small intestine is disordered.

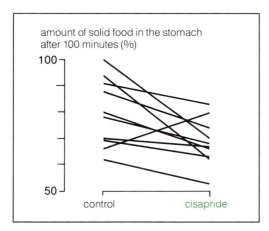

amount of solid food in the stomach
after 100 minutes (%)

100

50

control   cisapride·

*Figure 118: Cisapride accelerates
gastric emptying of solid food in
myotonic dystrophy, especially in those
patients with the slowest gastric
emptying. (Reproduced with
permission, from Horowitz et al., 1987a.)*

Prokinetics in myotonic dystrophy
It is important to recognise disordered
motility of the gastrointestinal tract in
patients with myotonic dystrophy since
they sometimes respond well to
cisapride (Figure 118). This drug
accelerates gastric emptying in these
patients, thereby reducing symptom
severity.

Conclusion

In systemic sclerosis, muscular
dystrophy and diabetes mellitus the
motility of stomach and intestines is often
diminished. The same picture (by
definition) applies to to CIIP. Prokinetics
that liberate acetylcholine (in particular
cisapride) are capable of stimulating
gastrointestinal motility, thereby
reducing symptom severity. In this way
the suffering of the patient is
considerably relieved.

References

Camilleri M, Brown ML, Malagelada JR. Impaired transit of chyme in chronic intestinal pseudoobstruction. Correction by cisapride. Gastroenterology 1986; 91: 619–626

Christensen J, Anuras S. Intestinal pseudoobstruction: Clinical features. In: Chey WY, ed. Functional disorders of the digestive tract. New York: Raven Press, 1983: 219–230

Feldman M, Smith HJ. Effect of cisapride on gastric emptying of indigestible solids in patients with gastroparesis diabeticorum. A comparison with metoclopramide and placebo. Gastroenterology 1987; 92: 171–174

Horowitz M, Maddox A, Wishart J, Collins PJ, Shearman DJC. Effects of cisapride on gastric and esophageal emptying in dystrophia myotonica. J Gastroenterol Hepatol 1987a; 2: 285–293

Horowitz M, Maddox A, Harding PE, e.a. Effects of cisapride on gastric and esophageal emptying in insulin-dependent diabetes mellitus. Gastroenterology 1987b; 92: 1899–1907

Horowitz M, Maddern GJ, Maddox A, Wishart J, Chatterton BE, Shearman DJC. Effects of cisapride on gastric and esophageal emptying in progressive systemic sclerosis. Gastroenterology 1987c; 93: 311–315

Hyser CL, Mendell JR. Recent advances in Duchenne and Becker muscular dystrophy. Neurol Clin 1988; 6: 429–453

Jozefowicz RF, Griggs RC. Myotonic dystrophy. Neurol Clin 1988; 6: 455–472

Kuhn E. Myotonische Dystrophie. In: Hopf HC, Poeck K, Schliack H, eds. Neurologie in Praxis und Klinik. Stuttgard: Georg Thieme, 1981: 1.82–1.88

Mortier W. Progressive Muskeldystrophien. In: Hopf HC, Poeck K, Schliack H, eds. Neurologie in Praxis und Klinik. Stuttgard: Georg Thieme, 1981: 1.34–1.62

Rowell NR. Lupus erythematosus, scleroderma and dermatomyositis. The "collagen" or "connective-tissue" diseases. In: Rook A, Wilkinson DS, Ebling FJG, Champion RH, Burton JL, eds. Textbook of dermatology. Oxford: Blackwell, 1986: 1281–1392

Smith B, The neuropathology of intestinal pseudo-obstruction. In: Chey WY, ed. Functional disorders of the digestive tract. New York: Raven Press. 1983: 231–236

Wehrmann T, Caspary WF. Einfluss von Cisaprid auf die Oesophagusmotilität bei Gesunden und Patienten mit progressiver systemischer Sklerodermie. Klin Wochtenschr 1990; 68: 602–607

Treatment

Chapter 14

Drug therapy

This chapter presents an overview of the major groups of drugs used to treat dysmotility

of the digestive tract.

Introduction

In recent years, the group of drugs which stimulate the movements of the gastrointestinal tract and control the secretion of gastric acid has been significantly extended. Thus, not only has progress been made in our knowledge of the physiology of the gastrointestinal tract and with regard to diagnostic techniques, but once a diagnosis has been made the disorder can be treated more rationally with more potent and more selective drugs.

Anti-acid drugs

Antacids

Even in ancient Rome, heartburn was treated with simple substances which chemically neutralized an acid stomach (so-called "antacids"). The idea behind this was very simple: complaints were attributed to the caustic gastric juices which were neutralized with the help of an alkaline agent. Indeed, gastric pH can be increased using an antacid agent. Within a few minutes of ingestion, the gastric pH rises, and it remains high for a considerable period thereafter (see Figure 119). Nowadays, a wide range of antacids is available, with various compositions. Antacids reduce the pain and heartburn which accompany ulcers and oesophagitis. On the other hand, it has not been demonstrated that they promote healing in gastric or duodenal ulcer or reflux oesophagitis. As far as functional (non-ulcerative) dyspepsia is concerned, they can provide short-term relief from symptoms that may be caused by gastric acid, but not from other symptoms, such as feeling of fullness or nausea.

Many of the antacids available today are combinations of magnesium and aluminium salts. These types of compounds are used because aluminium can cause constipation while magnesium has a laxative effect.

Now, with the advent of H_2-blockers (and omeprazole), drugs are available which have been shown to promote healing in oesophagitis and gastric or duodenal ulcer. This fact has led to a severe reduction in the use of antacids. Nevertheless, antacids continue to play a role. If patients with peptic ulcers or oesophagitis have an antacid within reach, they can use it to reduce occasional pain quickly and at will during treatment with H_2-blockers, prokinetic drugs or mucosal protectives.* Patients with mild, occasional, acid-related complaints (without ulcers or oesophagitis) can benifit from antacids used alone.

Histamine-H_2-blockers

Shortly after histamine was discovered, it became clear that it stimulated the secretion of gastric acid. However, the stimulation of gastric acid secretion was not influenced by the first antihistamines, which reduced the anaphylactic (allergic) effect of histamine. In 1972, a substance was made which reduced the effect of histamine on gastric acid, but not the allergic effect of histamine itself. It was called cimetidine. The only explanation of this phenomenon was the assumed presence of two distinct histamine receptors. The H_1-receptors play a role in allergy, whilst the H_2-receptors are involved in the secretion of gastric acid. Four different H_2-blockers are currently available for general use: cimetidine, ranitidine, nizatidine and famotidine.
Histamine-H_2-blockers were shown to be effective in the treatment of duodenal ulcers, gastric ulcers and oesophagitis. When these agents are used, gastric pH is increased for between 4 and 12 hours (Figure 119). It has been shown that H_2-blockers promote healing in ulcer and oesophagitis to a considerable extent.

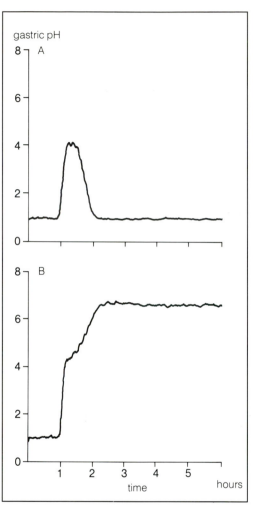

Figure 119: The gastric pH (as determined by pH monitoring) during antacid therapy. A: an antacid agent, algeldrate (10 ml); the rise in pH lasts about a half hour. B: An H_2-blocker, effervescent cimetidine (800 mg) with a buffer: the gastric pH is increased for several hours. (Reproduced with permission from Vlasblom et al., 1991.)

* Antacids reduce the uptake of cimetidine. It is recommended that no antacids be taken one hour before the ingestion of cimetidine.

Blocking H⁺/K⁺-ATPase

In the stomach, hydrochloric acid (HCl) is secreted by the parietal cells. The enzyme that secretes this HCl is called H^+/K^+-ATPase (the "proton pump"). Since 1990, omeprazole has been available; it inhibits the action of this enzyme in the parietal cells. In fact, omeprazole is a prodrug which is absorbed mainly by the parietal cells and is then converted (protonized) into a sulphonamide in the extremely acid environment around the parietal cells. This sulphonamide binds irreversibly with the H^+/K^+-ATPase and inhibits its action. Omeprazole greatly suppresses gastric acid production; at high doses, the secretion of acid is actually blocked completely. This makes it particularly suitable for severe disorders caused by gastric acid: gastric or duodenal ulcers which are severe or do not respond well to H_2-blockers, reflux oesophagitis (stage III and IV) and the Zollinger-Ellison syndrome. Omeprazole is more effective than H_2-blockers in the acute treatment of ulcers or severe oesophagitis.

Effects of antacid therapy

Gastric pH can be greatly increased for a considerable period using omeprazole and H_2-blockers. This promotes healing in ulcer and oesophagitis. However, raising the gastric pH also has other effects:

◆ When the gastric pH is increased by these drugs, the uptake of certain other drugs is altered. Many drugs and foods are less efficiently digested if the stomach is not acid*. With antacid therapy, drug secretion can also alter via the kidneys; for example, the plasma levels of salicylates may drop considerably, whilst those of quinidine rise.

◆ Gastric acid serves as a barrier to any living micro-organisms. Consequently, if it is neutralized, the likelihood of infection (e.g. through *Salmonella*) increases, particularly in groups at risk (old people or people with a weakened resistance).

The body has a regulatory system which endeavours to keep the stomach sufficiently acid: one consequence of all forms of antacid therapy is an action that tends to increase the production of gastric acid. This is achieved by gastrin: long-term, potent antacid therapy generally causes hypergastrinaemia. Severe hypergastrinaemia has been observed in animal experiments, but may be a matter of concern in humans, too.

---

* This applies to, amongst others, tetracyclines, isoniazide, quinidine, iron preparations, salicylates, ketoconazole, cimetidine, sodium fluoride (against tooth decay) and thiamine (vitamin B1)

Prokinetic drugs

Since the turn of the century, it has been known that the digestive tract is influenced by the sympathetic or parasympathetic nervous system. The sympathetic nervous system inhibits the movements and secretions of the digestive tract, and the parasympathetic nervous system stimulates them. From this knowledge it was a short step to initial ideas about drug therapy:

- the movements (and secretion) of the gastrointestinal tract should be stimulated by drugs that inhibit the sympathetic nervous system or enhance the functioning of the parasympathetic nervous system;
- the movements (and secretion) of the gastrointestinal tract should be inhibited by drugs that stimulate the sympathetic nervous system or inhibit the parasympathetic nervous system.

Adrenergic agonists do indeed reduce the movements of the gastrointestinal tract. And yet the development of adrenergic agonists or antagonists has not resulted in any clinically useable drugs which improve the movements of the gastrointestinal tract. Indeed, the movements of the gastrointestinal tract can probably be disturbed as a side-effect of adrenergic agonists or antagonists on the other hand, antagonists* of the dopamine-D_2-receptor are clinically useful for stimulating the movements of the gastrointestinal tract.

Dopamine-D_2-blockers

The discovery that neuroleptics reduce nausea and vomiting came more or less by chance, and the mechanism behind this was established rather quickly.

- The anti-emetic effect can be attributed to the blocking of dopamine-D_2-receptors. To achieve this it is (frequently) sufficient to block peripheral D_2-receptors. The blocking of D_2-receptors in the chemoreceptor trigger zone (which lies outside the blood-brain barrier) directly suppresses the sensation of nausea. Moreover, D_2-receptors in the stomach and duodenum are blocked, which stimulates gastric movements and gastroduodenal co-ordination and also reduces the chance of nausea. The anti-emetic effect depends partially on the prokinetic effect.
- With severe forms of vomiting, it may be desirable to block the D_2-receptors in the brain as well, so as to ensure an extremely powerful anti-emetic effect.

*We have in mind here clonidine, prazosin, propranolol and atenolol.

This was the reason why domperidone was developed. This substance is a peripherally-acting, selective D_2-blocker, which is used both as prokinetic and an anti-emetic drug. The D_2-blocker metoclopramide is also used as an anti-emetic. This substance does not merely block the D_2-receptors, but also (to a lesser extent) stimulates the release of acetylcholine. Metoclopramide has a peripheral and a central effect and, when it is used, one should be vigilant as to its central side-effects (extrapyramidal symptoms).

To suppress nausea and vomiting (e.g. in dyspepsia), domperidone is generally the treatment of choice, but for forms of nausea and vomiting (e.g. after chemotherapy, radiotherapy and operations) that do not readily respond to treatment, D_2-blockers, which also have a central effect, can be used, e.g. metoclopramide alizapride or a neuroleptic. If a neuroleptic is chosen, side-effects can best be avoided by use of a selective D_2-blocker, such as haloperidol, bromperidol, pimozide or sulpiride. Recently, new drugs have been introduced for the treatment of vomiting caused by chemotherapy: ondansetron and granisetron; these are (primarily) $5-HT_3$ antagonists.

Drugs which exert their effect via acetylcholine

The parasympathetic nervous system stimulates movements of the stomach and intestines, so it was common sense to stimulate peripheral cholinergic transmission with drugs in order to stimulate movements of the gastrointestinal tract. Intestinal atony used to be treated with the cholinergic receptor agonist, carbachol, and the cholinesterase inhibitors pyridostigmine and neostigmine. However, these substances have many side-effects and only narrow therapeutic applications. Since 1990, it has been possible to stimulate the effect of acetylcholine in the gastrointestinal tract indirectly and potently in another way, for there is a potent prokinetic drug available—cisapride—which works by releasing acetylcholine. This substance has special characteristics.

◆ It selectively stimulates the release of acetylcholine and thus stimulates the movements of the oesophagus, stomach and intestines (this influence on the release of acetylcholine is indirect—see Intermezzo 30). Cisapride stimulates gastric and intestinal movements more potently than D₂-antagonists.

◆ It probably influences the release of acetylcholine in the myenteric plexus, thereby affecting the movements of the gastrointestinal tract, but (remarkably enough) does not simultaneously stimulate the release of acetylcholine in other systems. Thus, the secretion of saliva and gastric juice, which is regulated in the submucosal plexus and which is also subject to the influence of acetylcholine, is not affected by cisapride.

In clinical terms, cisapride is suitable for a broad range of disorders characterized by insufficient gastrointestinal motility:

— oesophagitis due to reduced clearance of the oesophagus
— oesophagitis due to pathological gastro-oesophageal reflux
— functional (non-ulcer) dyspepsia
— chronic idiopathic intestinal pseudo-obstruction (CIIP)
— secondary dysmotility of the oesophagus, stomach and duodenum (Chapter 13), for example in diabetes mellitus, systemic sclerosis, some forms of muscular dystrophy, post-surgical gastroparesis, and sometimes anorexia nervosa.

Cisapride probably has a positive effect on some forms of constipation, but this has not yet been sufficiently investigated. Cisapride reduces the entire range of dyspeptic symptoms (see Figure 120).

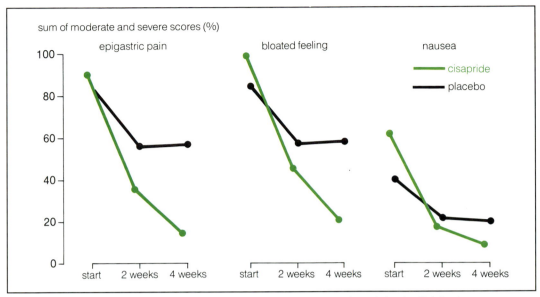

Figure 120: Cisapride (3 x 10 mg daily) reduces the severity of the individual symptoms of patients with functional (non-ulcer) dyspepsia. (Reproduced with permission, from Rösch et al., 1986.)

Intermezzo 30
The mechanism of action of cisapride

It quickly became clear that cisapride exerts its effect via the cholinergic system, because blocking the cholinergic transmission of muscarinic receptors (with atropine) cancelled out the effect of cisapride. For a long time it was unclear what the mechanism of action of cisapride was. It did not directly stimulate the acetylcholinergic receptors and (unlike the cholinesterase inhibitors) it did not inhibit the breakdown of acetylcholine. Further research led to the conclusion that cisapride, in one way or another, stimulated the release of acetylcholine. It did not act via any receptor which was known at the time (such as dopamine-D_2-, α- and β-adrenoreceptors, serotonin-5-HT_2-, histamine-H_1- and -H_2- and opiate μ-receptors). Recently, there have been indications that the effect of cisapride is primarily attributable to the activation of a newly discovered type of serotonin receptor, the 5-HT_4-receptor.
It is hypothesized that these receptors are preferentially (or indeed only) located on neurons in the myenteric plexus. This would explain the selective effect of cisapride on the gastrointestinal tract.

Mucosal protectives

For the treatment of gastric or duodenal ulcers, oesophagitis and erosive gastritis and duodenitis, use may be made of agents which protect the mucous membrane. In such cases, a choice may be made between two preparations:

◆ Sucralfate forms a complex with proteins on the mucous membrane, especially with injuries to the epithelium, and thus protects it against the gastric juices. Sucralfate is just about as effective as H_2-blockers and cisapride against oesophagitis (grade I and II) and combats peptic ulcers just as effectively as H_2-blockers. It is therefore used for peptic disorders of the oesophagus, stomach and duodenum.

◆ Bismuth subcitrate also forms a film over the ulcer, but it is generally used only to treat gastric and duodenal ulcers. It remains unclear whether bismuth subcitrate is also effective in the oesophagus. It also combats the bacterium *Helicobacter pylori*, although therapy with bismuth subcitrate completely eliminates this bacterium in only 20–30% of patients. It is still unclear whether the clinical effectiveness of bismuth subcitrate is primarily due to the protection of the mucous membrane or the eradication of *Helicobacter pylori*.

In severe cases of oesophagitis or in the treatment of gastric or duodenal ulcers, it is sensible to combine the use of mucosal protectives with other drugs (cisapride, H_2-blockers or omeprazole).

Smooth muscle relaxants

There are four distinct groups of drugs which relax the smooth muscle of the gastrointestinal tract.

Anticholinergic spasmolytics
Since the parasympathetic nervous system stimulates the gastrointestinal tract, it seemed logical to suppress spasms using muscarinic blockers ("anticholinergic agents", parasympatholytic agents). Here, we distinguish between drugs with and without a central effect. No central effect is anticipated with oxyphenonium and butyl scopolamine. Central (side-)effects are observed with the use of atropine.

Other spasmolytics
In addition, there are spasmolytics, such as pinaverium and mebeverine, which act directly on smooth muscle. These substances are used to treat colonic spasms (in painful IBS).

Nitrates
Nitrates have traditionally been used mainly to treat heart complaints. Nitroglycerine, isosorbide dinitrate, pentaerythritol tetranitrate, and related substances are available. However, these drugs can also be used to treat oesophageal spasms and dyskinesia of the sphincter of Oddi. The use of these agents is based on clinical experience; their effectiveness in patients suffering from gastrointestinal complaints has not yet been fully investigated.

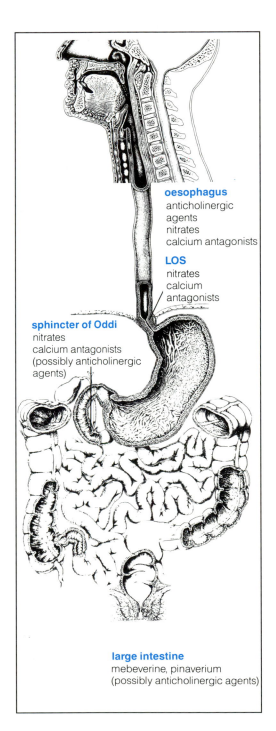

Calcium antagonists

For the contraction of smooth muscle cells it is important that calcium ions can flow in through calcium channels. However, some substances (socalled calcium antagonists) keep these calcium channels closed. Examples are nifedipine, verapamil and diltiazem. Calcium antagonists are often used to treat spasms and other oesophageal motility disorders as well as dyskinesia of the sphincter of Oddi. The use of these agents is based on clinical experience; their effectiveness in patients suffering from gastrointestinal complaints has not yet been fully investigated.

How to choose a smooth muscle relaxant?

Figure 121 shows the locations in the gastrointestinal tract for which individual smooth muscle relaxants are primarily used. The applications presented are based mainly on practical experience in the use of these drugs, rather than on the basis of good comparative trials. These data are also summarized in Table 13 (see p. 269).

oesophagus
anticholinergic
agents
nitrates
calcium antagonists

LOS
nitrates
calcium
antagonists

sphincter of Oddi
nitrates
calcium antagonists
(possibly anticholinergic
agents)

large intestine
mebeverine, pinaverium
(possibly anticholinergic agents)

Figure 121: Overview of the locations in the gastrointestinal tract in which individual smooth muscle relaxants are used.

Laxatives

Laxatives may be indicated in (genuine) cases of constipation, especially if the results obtained by fibre-enrichment of the food are unsatisfactory (Intermezzo 31). There are various groups of laxatives.

◆ Volume-increasing laxatives. Extra dietary fibre may be taken in the form of bulking agents, such as psyllium seed or sterculia gum. Fibre increases the volume of the faecal material and retains water. Furthermore, bacteria can completely digest these fibres, so that dietary fibre increases the volume of bacteria in the faeces.

◆ Osmotic laxatives. These may be used to make faecal material looser and more liquid. To achieve this, a choice can be made between simple salts, e.g. magnesium compounds (magnesium oxide, sulphate or citrate), lactulose or a lactulose analogue, lactitol.

◆ Contact laxatives act on the mucous membrane of the large intestine, stimulating extra contractions therein. These laxatives include bisacodyl and enemas with soap and phosphate. There is reluctance to use senna preparations, as they probably damage the myenteric plexus of the colon if used for a prolonged period.

Intermezzo 31
The effect of dietary fibre

The importance of dietary fibre is generally emphasized for normal defaecation. Some dietary fibres are not broken down totally, not even by intestinal bacteria, whilst others (e.g. pectins) are. Some fibres retain a large quantity of water (e.g. brans) and others retain very little or none at all.

Is dietary fibre really important for defaecation?
Dietary fibre increases faecal volume and makes faeces less solid. However, it has not been demonstrated that constipation in patients is due to their eating insufficient dietary fibre. Dietary fibre mostly has a positive effect on constipation, although this effect is not always sufficient. Most placebo-controlled trials have failed to show a clearly beneficial effect of dietary fibre on pain in IBS. For the time being, the available data do not point to any single, clear conclusion. There may well be a sub-group of IBS patients suffering pain who are helped by dietary fibre, but this sub-group has not yet been sufficiently characterized. In fact, the trial results were probably negative because the group of patients examined was too heterogeneous. It is also known that, besides its positive effects, dietary fibre has negative effects (gas formation, feeling of fullness). This may explain why the net effect of the treatment was not clearly positive.

Most patients are sufficiently relieved by short-term laxative treatment, but it is sometimes necessary to use laxatives for a prolonged period (even for life).

Antidiarrhoeal drugs

There are many examples of relatively innocuous infectious disease that can cause acute diarrhoea. In these cases, great efforts to make accurate diagnoses are not justified. The body has sufficient protection against such infections, and it may be the case that the bacterium or virus in question has already been sufficiently combatted by the time the doctor examines the patient. However, in order to spare the patient the discomfort of diarrhoea, a symptomatic approach is often required.

There is nothing new about the constipatory and antidiarrhoeal effect of opium (and morphine). Old antidiarrhoeal drugs (opium tincture with saffron) were based on them, but these are now obsolete due to their side-effects and the risk of addiction. At present there is actually only one suitable agent for the symptomatic treatment of diarrhoea: loperamide. This controls diarrhoea mainly by stimulating peripheral opiate receptors.* It also blocks calcium channels, and this may also contribute to the antidiarrhoeal effect. Moreover, it reduces intestinal movements and probably stimulates the resorption of water and electrolytes. Oral rehydration (oral rehydration salts, ORS) is recommended for children suffering from diarrhoea. In many countries, the traditional treatment of diarrhoea still involves activated charcoal, but it has not been demonstrated that this agent either reduces or shortens the duration of diarrhoea, although it may be used as a remedy in the treatment of intoxication.

* Loperamide is so effectively converted by the liver that no central opiate effects are observed (except in children under 2 years old, for whom it is consequently not indicated).

Conclusion: a selection of drugs

The use of drugs to treat disturbed movements of the digestive tract is summarized in Table 13. We shall discuss this briefly below, taking one disorder at a time.

Reflux-related complaints and reflux oesophagitis

In the treatment of reflux-related complaints or reflux oesophagitis, distinctions are made depending on the gravity of the disorder and the use of acute or maintenance treatment.

◆ Patients complaining of relatively mild heartburn, without oesophagitis being diagnosed, may be treated with prokinetic drugs, antacids, or both. If the complaints persist, an H_2-blocker may be administered for a few weeks.

◆ For the acute treatment of oesophagitis (stages I and II), a choice may be made between cisapride, H_2-blockers or sucralfate; these drugs have a roughly equivalent effect. Combining these drugs increases the chances of healing. It may also be possible to use omeprazole, but most specialists currently reserve this agent for more severe or therapy-resistant forms of oesophagitis. In fact, it is logical to use a prokinetic drug, since dysmotility is often involved in reflux oesophagitis.

◆ For the acute treatment of oesophagitis (stages III and IV), there is a choice between omeprazole, or a combination of cisapride and a high dose of an H_2-blocker, sucralfate sometimes being added to this combination.

◆ In order that relapse should be prevented, oesophagitis often requires maintenance treatment. The effect of maintenance treatment with a conventional dose of an H_2-blocker is disappointing, but when used in high doses, H_2-blockers probably lower the chances of relapse. There are indications that low-dose cisapride may be effective in preventing relapse. The use of a prokinetic drug is also more logical than prolonged treatment with H_2-blockers. In some patients with serious relapse, there is no alternative but to opt for maintenance treatment with omeprazole.

Functional (non-ulcer) dyspepsia

Delayed gastric emptying is a frequent symptom of functional dyspepsia. This may be treated with prokinetic drugs, i.e. D_2-blockers or prokinetic drugs that release acetylcholine. Prokinetic drugs are highly suitable for reducing the symptoms of functional dyspepsia. If nausea or vomiting predominate, there is a tendency to use a D_2-blocker, or otherwise a prokinetic drug that releases acetylcholine. Among prokinetic drugs, cisapride has the strongest effect.

Gastric or duodenal ulcers

Various forms of treatment are possible for gastric and duodenal ulcers. The most frequent choice involves the use of an H_2-blocker or omeprazole to reduce the secretion of gastric acid. Ulcers may also be treated with sucralfate or

	antacid therapy (1)	prokinetic drugs (2)	mucosal protective drugs (3)	smooth muscle relaxants (4)	laxatives	antidiarrhoeal drugs (5)
oesophageal dysmotility						
— spasms				AS, N, Caa		
— hypoperistalsis		cis, met, dom				
— achalasia of the LOS				AS, N, Caa		
reflux complaints	A, H₂-	cis, met, dom				
reflux oesophagitis:						
— acute, stage I, II	H₂-, (om)	cis	suc			
— acute, stage III, IV	om, (H₂-)	(cis)	suc			
— maintenance treatment		cis				
dyspepsia						
— pain due to gastric acid	A	cis, met, dom				
— nausea, vomiting		dom, met				
— delayed gastric emptying		cis, met, dom				
gastric or duodenal ulcer	om, H₂-		suc, bis			
Zollinger-Ellison syndrome	om					
dyskinesia of the sphincter of Oddi				N, Caa (AS)		
paralytic ileus		cis				
enteroparesis		cis				
IBS						
— mainly diarrhoea						lop
— mainly constipation		(cis)			+	
— spasms				M/P, (AS)		
severe constipation		(cis)			+	
CIIP		cis				
secondary dysmotility		cis				

1. A = antacids
   H₂- = H₂-blockers
   om = omeprazole
2. cis = cisapride
   dom = domperidone
   met = metoclopramide
3. bis = bismuth subcitrate
   suc = sucralfate
4. AS = anticholinergic spasmolytics
   Caa = calcium antagonists
   M/P = mebeverine/pinaverium
   N = nitrates
5. lop = loperamide

Table 13: Overview of which drugs are suitable for particular disorders.

bismuth subcitrate. H_2-blockers are mainly used for maintenance treatment. This reduces the percentage of patients suffering relapse.

The distal digestive tract

The movements of the proximal digestive tract have been studied far more extensively than those of the small and large intestines. This applies not merely to normal movements, but also to dysmotility. It is anticipated that there will soon be some ideas about the diagnosis and treatment of disturbances in the distal digestive tract, which are better supported by empirical findings. Table 13 gives a current overview of the drugs used to treat disorders of the small and large intestines.

References

Rösch H. Cisapride in non-ulcer dyspepsia. Scand J Gastroenterol 1986; 104: 544

Vlasblom V e.a. Effects of a new effervescent cimetidine formulation on gastric acidity in healthy subjects. Neth J Med 1991; 38: 147–152

Chapter 15

Surgery

Some gastrointestinal motility disorders can be rectified by means of surgery. But surgery can also disrupt motility patterns. This chapter briefly discusses the most important operations.

Longitudinal oesophageal myotomy

Oesophageal spasms can cause severe, and sometimes even debilitating, pain, which cannot always be adequately controlled by the use of drugs. In such cases, one often performs a longitudinal oesophageal myotomy. This involves making a longitudinal incision 10 cm long in a part of the oesophageal muscle layer, as deep as the mucosa. If the oesophagus contracts spastically after surgery, the pressure in the oesophagus and the oesophageal tension cannot rise to pre-surgical levels. Oesophageal spasms are mostly less painful after this operation.

Heller's myotomy

In achalasia (of the LOS), pneumatic dilation of the LOS is considered the treatment of choice*. However, this treatment is not always successful, and is best not performed on a patient with an oesophageal diverticulum. In such a case, one can proceed to myotomy of the LOS (Heller's myotomy). In this operation, a longitudinal incision several centimetres long is made in the LOS, as far as the mucous membrane. This procedure greatly reduces the pressure in the LOS and greatly enhances passage through it. A certain amount of precision is required so as not to cut through too much or too little of the muscle layer. If the surgeon transects the muscle layer insufficiently, the achalasia will remain. To prevent this, manometry of the LOS is often carried out during the operation. In this way, the extent to which the surgery has lowered the pressure in the LOS can be seen during the operation itself. In most cases, the muscles are cut through until the pressure in the LOS has disappeared. If this pressure drops to zero, there is a distinct possibility of reflux. That is why Heller's myotomy is often combined with an anti-reflux operation (mostly Nissen fundoplication). However, it has not yet been thoroughly investigated whether peroperative manometry on the one hand and the combination of Heller's myotomy and Nissen's anti-reflux procedure on the other are clearly beneficial.

* In achalasia, nitrates or calcium antagonists offer an alternative form of treatment. Since these agents are only occasionally effective, pneumatic dilation is considered to be the treatment of choice.

Anti-reflux procedures

Some patients suffering from recurrent severe reflux oesophagitis require surgical treatment (p. 84). There are various surgical techniques for controlling gastro-oesophageal reflux (Table 4, p. 82), but since the introduction of H_2-blockers, fewer and fewer of these operations have been performed. The introduction of an Angelchick prosthesis (a silicon rubber ring placed around the cardia) has been abandoned due to the large number of (sometimes serious) complications. At present, most of the surgery performed is done according to Nissen's procedure (Figure 122). In this operation, the uppermost part of the stomach is folded like a collar around the LOS. The operation can result in an impressive reduction of reflux, and in many cases the reflux of gastric contents into the oesophagus stops completely. However, anti-reflux operations quite often result in complications, some of which are irreversible. Serious complications arise in particular through unintentional damage to the vagus nerve. For this reason, anti-reflux operations are always based on strict indications and contraindications (with the aid of pH-monitoring, manometry and a gastric emptying study, see p. 84). Previously, the diagnosis of patients with reflux complaints was often based exclusively on an X-ray. Today, better indications and improved surgical techniques have resulted in a higher success rate and a longer-lasting effectiveness of surgery.

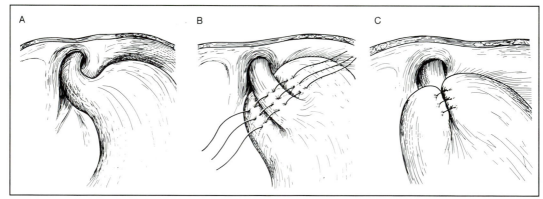

Figure 122: Nissen fundoplication. In this procedure the fundus of the stomach is wrapped like a collar around the LOS.

Vagotomies

A truncal or selective vagotomy can be performed in order to prevent recurrence of peptic ulcers, although its performance is sometimes the unintended consequence of another operation. After a truncal vagotomy, there is no adaptive relaxation of the proximal stomach (p. 90), which causes relatively high intra-abdominal pressure after eating or drinking. This, in turn, results in accelerated gastric emptying of liquids. After a truncal or selective vagotomy, the stomach produces too few movements. This results in delayed gastric emptying of solids. In many cases, the symptoms are so severe that pyloroplasty is required to accelerate the passage of the gastric contents (Figure 123). However, this does not always help, and pyloroplasty is less effective if gastric emptying is primarily delayed due to suppressed antral mixing and grinding movements. Current practice most frequently entails the use of highly selective vagotomy (HSV), in which the branches of the vagus leading to the corpus and fundus are severed, but not those leading to the antrum and pylorus. This procedure denervates the acid-forming part of the stomach, but not the motor part. HSV gives better results than other vagotomies, but may also give rise to complications. If these respond insufficiently to conservative treatment, a Roux-en-Y operation can be considered. Should gastric emptying be too slow after the vagotomy, a prokinetic drug that releases acetylcholine may be prescribed.

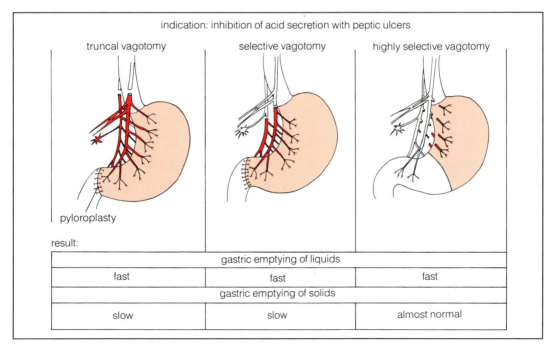

Figure 123: The various gastric vagotomies with their indications and consequences for gastric emptying.

Operations on the stomach and proximal small intestine

Stomach surgery is necessary for the treatment of gastric carcinoma and sometimes also useful for treating severe, recurrent peptic ulcers. H_2-blockers often provide a good alternative to resection of the stomach in many cases. The most frequently performed stomach operations are Billroth partial gastrectomies (Figure 124).

Billroth I (B-I) partial gastrectomy entails the removal of the pylorus and part of the distal stomach; the remainder of the stomach is then connected to the duodenum. Billroth II (B-II) partial gastrectomy results in the gastric contents emptying into the jejunum instead of into the duodenum. After both B-I and B-II partial gastrectomies, the stomach is sometimes emptied so fast that "dumping" arises. B-II partial gastrectomy sometimes results in delayed gastric emptying of a solid meal. Furthermore, bile can easily enter the stomach after this operation, which may result in bilious vomiting. In some cases, these complications are so serious that an additional operation, Roux-en-Y reconstruction, must be performed. The intestinal loop, along with the bile ducts, duodenum and proximal jejunum, receives a new opening into the small intestine which is more distal to the gastric outlet. This Roux-en-Y reconstruction is also performed to remedy gastric emptying disorders following a highly selective vagotomy (HSV, p. 275). Roux-en-Y reconstruction can often suppress bilious vomiting and "dumping". However, an occasional complication arising from this operation is that stasis may occur in the part of the jejunum connecting the stomach to the remainder of the small intestine (the so-called "Roux loop"). Some patients still suffer from delayed gastric emptying after the Roux-en-Y operation (the so-called Roux-en-Y syndrome).

Delayed gastric emptying after a Billroth-II or Roux-en-Y partial gastrectomy may also be treated with prokinetic drugs that release acetylcholine. The effect of this therapy has not yet been systematically investigated in a sufficiently large group of patients, but the first provisional results of treatment using cisapride are encouraging, as had been anticipated in view of its mechanism of action.

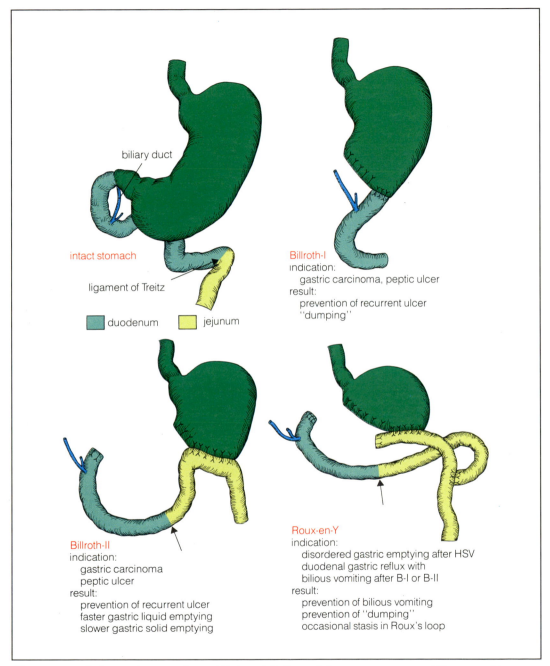

biliary duct

intact stomach

ligament of Treitz

duodenum   jejunum

Billroth-I
indication:
    gastric carcinoma, peptic ulcer
result:
    prevention of recurrent ulcer
    "dumping"

Billroth-II
indication:
    gastric carcinoma
    peptic ulcer
result:
    prevention of recurrent ulcer
    faster gastric liquid emptying
    slower gastric solid emptying

Roux-en-Y
indication:
    disordered gastric emptying after HSV
    duodenal gastric reflux with
    bilious vomiting after B-I or B-II
result:
    prevention of bilious vomiting
    prevention of "dumping"
    occasional stasis in Roux's loop

Figure 124: Schematic overview of B-I and B-II partial gastrectomy and Roux-en-Y reconstruction with their indications and their consequences for gastric emptying.

Investigation techniques

Chapter 16

Techniques for the investigation of the movements of the gastrointestinal tract

A whole range of investigation techniques can be used to study motility disorders of the gastrointestinal tract and their consequences. The most important of these are briefly described here.

Radiography

Radiography is the oldest and best-tested method of examining internal organs non-invasively. Although many investigation techniques have now been introduced, radiography is essential for answering a number of questions. However, radiology has one distinct disadvantage when it comes to studying the movements of parts of the gastrointestinal tract: the dose of radiation it delivers makes prolonged observations inadmissible. Although a special dynamic technique called cineradiography is often performed (e.g. in swallow and defaecation disorders), methods of dynamic investigation (such as ultrasonography, manometry, pH monitoring or scintigraphy) that involve smaller doses of radiation are to be preferred.

Radiography with barium contrast
If part of the intestine is filled with barium paste, the walls of the part of the intestine of interest can be made visible on X-ray. If air (gas) is used in addition to barium paste the radiopaque liquid sticks to the wall, while the radiolucent air fills the lumen, giving a double contrast. This procedure often provides clearer images (cf. Figure 79, p. 152). Using radiography with a barium paste or double contrast, the entire gastrointestinal tract (from the mouth to the anus) may be studied.
Radiography is primarily important for excluding organic disorders (stenosis) and establishing the existence of a widening (dilation) which may be the result of a motility disorder.

Endoscopic retrograde cholangiopancreaticography (ERCP)

ERCP is a special radiographic technique used to make the bile ducts and the pancreatic ducts visible*. A flexible, fibre-optic endoscope is introduced into the duodenum, and the papilla of Vater is cannulated via the instrumentation channel. Then, a contrast medium is injected into the bile ducts and the pancreatic duct. Subsequently, these passages can be seen on the X-ray (see Figure 55, p. 117) and any dilation of the common bile duct can be shown. The patient is mostly sedated for this examination.

Plain film of the abdomen
It is possible by means of an X-ray to distinguish between liquids, gases and faecal material in the intestines without use of a contrast media. This is particularly important when an ileus is suspected. For if a (pseudo-)obstruction of the intestines is suspected, one will certainly not want to place a burden on the gastrointestinal tract by using a contrast medium. If the patient is lying down, the expanded intestinal loops may be observed; if he is standing, the air fluid levels in the intestines can be seen (Figure 72, p. 141). A plain film of the abdomen may also be used to assess the degree of faecal accumulation in the colon in patients suffering from constipation. Thus, in both applications of a plain film of the abdomen it is the consequences of dysmotility which are observed, rather than the movements themselves.

---

* One complication of ERCP is pancreatitis (in approximately 1% of the patients examined).

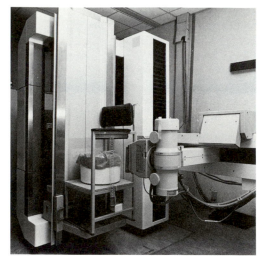

Figure 125: Set-up for defaecography. (Reproduced with permission, from Dr R. Goei, Heerlen.)

Defaecography

Defaecography is a form of cineradiography designed to make the defecation process visible. The rectum is filled with a contrast medium which has the same volume and viscosity as normal faeces. The patient sits on an inflated rubber tyre (which permits the passage of X-rays, see Figure 125). By means an X-ray camera, a film can then be made of the actual defaecation process. A film of this kind demonstrates the movements of the rectum, anal canal and pelvic floor during defaecation. Attention is paid to the following symptoms in the resting, squeezing and straining state:
— the anorectal angle,
— lowering of the pelvic floor,
— anatomical changes during squeezing, straining and defaecation (e.g. rectocoele, prolapse and intussusception),

— the length and diameter of the anal canal,
— the opening of the anal canal,
— the expulsion of the contrast medium.

Pellet passage test

The speed of passage through the gastrointestinal tract can be measured by having the patient swallow pellets or rings which can then be monitored on X-ray pictures (Figure 126). The mouth to anus transit time is normally 1–3 days. Of this period, the passage from the mouth into the large intestine accounts for 1–6 hours. In practice, the (radiographic) pellet passage test is rarely used to measure transport through the stomach and small intestine, but is applied for transport through the large intestine. Passage is said to be delayed if, after 4 days, 4 or more of the 20 pellets are still in the intestines. If the particles remain in the large intestine for too long, the diagnosis of constipation is objectively confirmed and, what is more, one can see where the pellets are located in the colon. Comparable information may be obtained by scintigraphy.

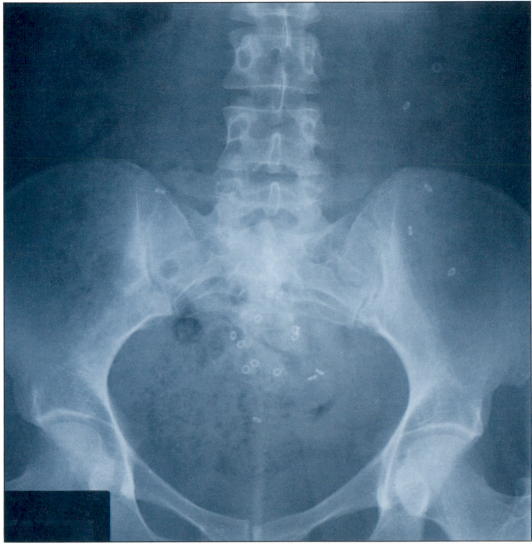

Figure 126: X-ray of the intestines of a patient who has ingested radiopaque rings so that colon transit time can be measured.

Scintigraphy

There are various ways of introducing radioactive tracers into the gastrointestinal tract in order to study their transport. The great advantage of scintigraphy is that transit through the gastrointestinal tract can be observed for prolonged periods using a technique which places little strain on the patient (Figure 127).

Furthermore, with scintigraphy, the properties of the test meals can be altered systematically, although scintigraphy does not provide the same resolution as radiography. Moreover, there is no need to use non-physiological contrast media.

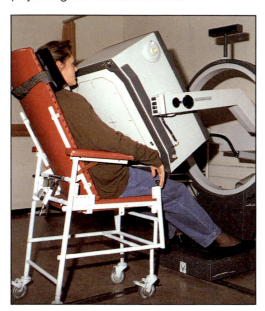

Figure 127: Photograph of the set-up for scintigraphic examination using a scintillation camera.

Gastric emptying studies

Scintigraphy is the technique used for gastric emptying studies. In fact, it is now considered to be the standard test for this purpose. The technique displays the stomach and its movements, as well as the duodenum, with exceptional clarity (Figure 128). A whole range of test meals is used, ranging from liquid to solid.

In most cases, the radioactive tracer ^{99m}Technetium is used, which has a half-life of 6 hours. Another substance used is the isotope ^{113}Indium, which has a half-life of 1.5 hours. Gastric liquid and solid emptying can be studied during a single experiment. The liquid meal is labelled with ^{113}Indium, which is coupled to diethylene triaminopenta-acetic acid

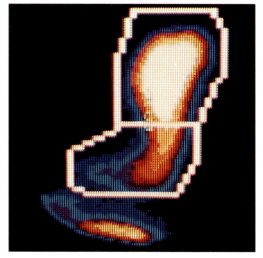

Figure 128: The result of scintigraphy. Here we see the stomach and a portion of the duodenum. The scintigraphic image is transposed into colour codes (blue means low radioactivity, red more, yellow even more and white most of all. (Reproduced with permission, from Dr M. Horowitz, Adelaide.)

(DTPA) and the solid meal is labelled with ^{99m}Technetium, which is coupled to a tin colloid. Both isotopes can be separately monitored by a scintillation camera; then gastric emptying and intestinal filling can be measured over time (cf. Figure 41, p. 96).

HIDA scintigraphy

Special tracers can be used to observe bile transport, for example iminodiacetic acid (IDA) and its analogues. These substances are selectively and efficiently filtered out of the blood by the liver and excreted into the bile. It is preferable to use dimethyl-IDA, which is radioactively labelled (often with ^{99m}Technetium), and which is administered to patients intravenously. Bile transport can be monitored using a scintillation camera (just as with gastric emptying studies). This method is called HIDA scan (hepatobiliary IDA). Using the HIDA scan it was discovered, amongst other things, that normally, in healthy individuals, some of the duodenal contents flow back into the stomach.

Measurement of transport through the small intestine

Scintigraphic examination of the small intestine is performed in the same way as for the stomach. The patient ingests a radioactively marked test meal, and the progress of this meal through the gastrointestinal tract is monitored with the help of a scintillation camera. The moment at which the first radioactivity arrives in the caecum can usually be accurately determined. Abnormalities in the passage through the small intestine are more accurately established by scintigraphy than by radiography. The effect of drugs on the passage of food through the small intestine can also be accurately assessed by means of scintigraphy.

Measurement of transport through the large intestine

In order to measure transport through the large intestine, a radioactive material is introduced into the right colon using a catheter or specially coated tablets, and then monitored (cf. Figure 82, p. 154). However, this is still an experimental technique.

Measurement of transport through the entire gastrointestinal tract

Recent research has focused on transport through the entire gastrointestinal tract, using radio-labelled plastic particles. These particles measure less than 1 mm across (and can therefore pass through the pylorus in the fed state, cf. p. 100) and are homogeneously mixed with the food. Gastric emptying and transport through segments of the small and large intestines can be followed using a scintillation camera.

Manometry

Manometry of the gastrointestinal tract has considerably extended our knowledge of the movements of this organ system. The same claim can be made for virtually all parts of the gastrointestinal tract. We now know a great deal about the normal movements of most parts of the gastrointestinal tract and manometry is an important tool for detecting motility disorders. Only in the case of the large intestine are the normal movements still poorly understood, so manometry of the large intestine is still a research technique.

Open-tip catheters and mini transducers

For some time now, the manometric technique has incorporated a catheter with various lumina, each of which is connected to a pressure sensor and perfused with water. The perfusion flow is constant (0.2–0.3 ml/min) and is independent of the pressure in the lumen. Outside the body, the pressure in the system is transformed into an electrical signal. At present, instead of perfused catheters, catheters with mini transducers are also used (Figure 129). These sensors transform the pressure in the body into an electrical signal. This makes it unnecessary to have a system

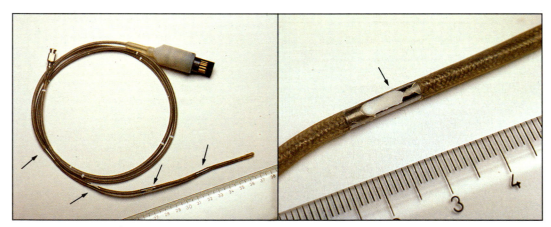

Figure 129: Catheter with mini transducers (arrows) for manometric studies.

which continuously pumps a strictly controlled flow of water through the catheter. Thanks to the mini transducers, prolonged manometric examinations can be performed on out-patients. If the pressure of a sphincter is to be measured, the catheter can be pulled slowly through the sphincter while the pressure is measured ("pull-through profile"). Super-thin catheters (e.g. 1.7 mm) can be used for special purposes (e.g. manometry of the sphincter of Oddi).

Manometry of sphincters with the Dent sleeve

The problem with conventional manometry is that pressure can only be measured very locally. Also, prolonged measurement of the pressure of a sphincter poses a problem. Sometimes, a small movement of the catheter means that suddenly, instead of measuring the

pressure of the sphincter, one measures the pressure of the distal or proximal part of the intestine. In 1976, Dent developed a sensor with a thin silicon rubber membrane under which water is perfused (Figure 130). The sensor measures the highest pressure exerted on the membrane, making it possible to obtain reliable prolonged measurements of sphincteric pressure. A short or long membrane is used, depending on the sphincter of interest. For manometry of the LOS a membrane 5–6 cm long is usually used.

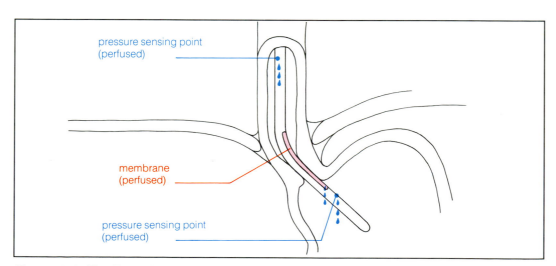

pressure sensing point (perfused)

membrane (perfused)

pressure sensing point (perfused)

Figure 130: The Dent sleeve.

Endoscopy

The advent of the flexible endoscope has enabled many studies which are required for valid diagnostics. The diagnosis of oesophagitis is best established using endoscopic images, while the same applies for gastric and duodenal erosions and ulcers. Colonoscopy is the prime technique for observing inflammations, stenoses or tumours in the colon. Endoscopy is not only important for showing up abnormalities; the instrumentation channel of a flexible endoscope can be used to perform a broad range of manoeuvres in the body, obtain a biopsy, remove a polyp or introduce a catheter containing a pressure sensor. Endoscopy is not the most suitable method for monitoring the motility disorders themselves as gastric and intestinal motor activities are influenced in a non-physiological manner. Furthermore, this form of examination is trying for the patient, making prolonged recordings out of the question.

The breath hydrogen test

The small intestine in humans is unable to break down and resorb some carbohydrates (e.g. stachyose from beans or synthetic lactulose). Bacteria in the large intestine can metabolize these carbohydrates, releasing gaseous hydrogen in the process (see Figure 131). This hydrogen finds its way into the blood and is exhaled. By administering a test meal containing non-resorbable carbohydrates and measuring the concentration of hydrogen in the exhaled breath, we can ascertain how long it takes for food to reach the caecum. If there is bacterial overgrowth in the stomach or small intestine, there will be an unexpectedly early peak in the hydrogen curve. Using the breath hydrogen test alone, it is impossible to distinguish bacterial overgrowth from accelerated transit through the stomach and small intestine. Combining the breath hydrogen test with radiographic or scintigraphic examination of the transit time enables this distinction; if there is a peak in the hydrogen curve, the exact location of the tracers can be observed.

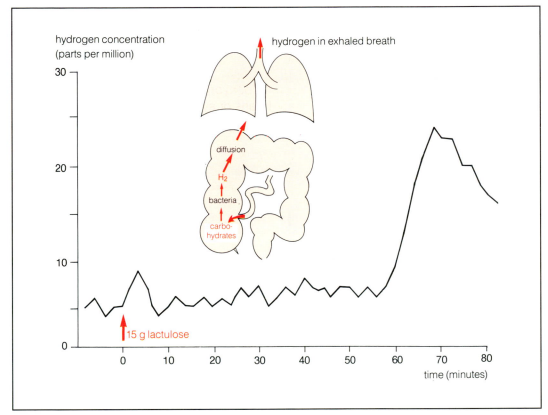

Figure 131: Measurement of the speed of transit through the small intestine with the breath hydrogen test. The diagram illustrates the principle of the technique. In the graph, 15 g of lactulose has been administered, and after about 70 minutes there is a sudden rise in the quantity of hydrogen in the exhaled breath. This is the time at which the lactulose arrives in the caecum.

Ultrasonography

Forming images with ultrasound is a fairly recent and an easily applicable technique for studying the internal organs non-invasively. The movements of the stomach, pylorus and duodenum can be readily observed after the subject drinks about 300 ml of liquid (Figure 132). If ultrasonograms are studied on a screen for about 15 minutes, an idea of the contraction profile of the antrum or pylorus and the proximal duodenum can be obtained. Furthermore, a relationship can be established between the contractions of the antrum, pylorus and duodenum on the one hand and the flow through the pylorus on the other. Ultrasound makes it possible to make more or less quantitative measurements of gastric liquid emptying. However, such an examination requires great experience and has consequently only been used until now for research purposes. Ultrasonography can also be used to make direct observations of gallbladder emptying. Postprandial gallbladder emptying is induced by means of a fatty meal, a bar of chocolate, or intravenous administration of CCK8 ("pancreozymin") or ceruletide. If recordings are made from two directions, the volume of the gallbladder can be determined (Figure 58, p. 121). This also makes it possible to observe the (minor) interdigestive gallbladder emptying.

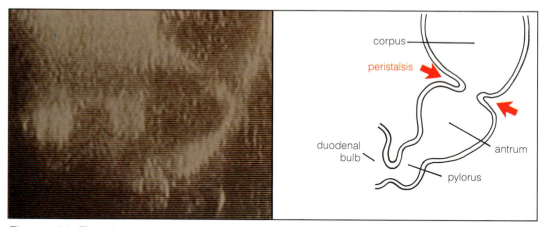

Figure 132: The ultrasonographic image of the antrum, pylorus and duodenum after the subject has drunk the fluid.

pH monitoring

Using a miniature pH electrode on a flexible catheter, it is possible to monitor measurements of oesophageal or gastric pH over a prolonged period (24 hours). Twenty-four-hour pH monitoring is the proper method for diagnosing gastro-oesophageal reflux. The thin catheter is inserted through the nose (Figure 133). In the oesophagus, this electrode is positioned 5 cm above the LOS. The catheter is then fastened to the nose and linked up to a portable recorder and the patient is sent home with the recorder attached to a belt round his or her waist. During the monitoring period the patient can indicate, by pressing a button on the recorder, whenever a symptom becomes bothersome. Gastric pH can also easily be monitored, although the clinical value of such a procedure is not yet entirely clear. In scientific research, gastric pH can be monitored in an attempt to quantify the effect of antacids or inhibitors of gastric acid secretion.

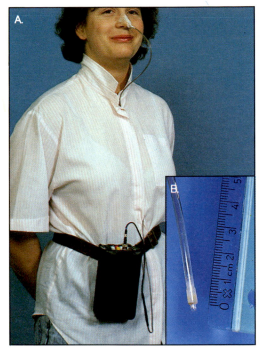

Figure 133: A: A catheter bearing a pH electrode is inserted through the nose and positioned at the correct location; the signals it picks up are recorded over 24 hours on a portable recorder.
B: A pH electrode for 24 hour pH monitoring in ambulatory persons. The type of electrode shown here is made of glass and has a built-in reference electrode.

Electromyographic techniques

Muscle cell contractions are accompanied by changes in electrical potential across the membrane. These changes can be registered using electrodes. Three totally different methods are pertinent to the study of the gastrointestinal tract:
— electrogastrography (EGG): study of the electrical control activity of the smooth muscle cells of the stomach;
— electromyography (EMG) of the smooth muscle cells of the oesophagus, small and large intestine and the internal anal sphincter;

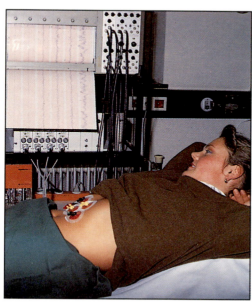

Figure 134 Recording equipment for electrogastrography (EGG).

— electromyography of the external anal sphincter and the muscles of the pelvic floor.

Electrogastrography (EGG)
The electrical activity in the stomach (ECA and ERA) can be measured by means of electrodes that are placed on the upper abdomen (Figure 134). When these data have been analysed, an overview of the electrical control activity is obtained. It is observed that the frequency drops slightly after a meal and then rises again (Figure 135). In this way, irregularities or changes of frequency of this electrical control activity (dysrhythmia, tachygastria) can be established.

Electromyography of the smooth muscle
For research purposes, this method can be used to record the electrical activity of smooth muscles in all parts of the gastrointestinal tract. The electrodes can be applied to the mucosa from the intestinal lumen or (during surgery) from the outside of the intestine near the muscle layer. In this way, a record of both the electrical control activity and the action potentials of these muscle cells can be determined.

Electromyography of the striated muscle

Contractions of striated muscles are accompanied by action potentials. These action potentials can be recorded using extracellular electrodes (EMG). This technique is frequently used for examining striated muscles in the extremities. EMG can also be used to monitor the functioning of the external anal sphincter and the muscles of the pelvic floor (p. 192).

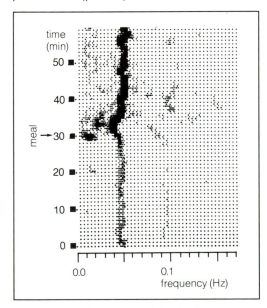

Figure 135: Gastric activity before and after a meal. Shown are the data obtained by means of an EGG analysis.

	radiology	scintigraphy	ultrasonography	endoscopy	manometry	pH monitoring	EGG	EMG of smooth muscle	EMG of striated muscle	breath hydrogen test
oesophagus:										
motility disorders	(+)	+			++			+		
stenosis, tumour	+			++						
pathological reflux						++				
oesophagitis				++						
stomach:										
gastroparesis					++					
stenosis, tumour, inflammation	+			++						
erosion, ulcer	+			++						
gastric dysrhythmia							++	++		
disturbed gastric emptying	(+)	++	+							
gallbladder and bile ducts:										
gall stones	++		++	+						
disturbed gallbladder emptying	+	+	++							
dyskinesia of sphincter of Oddi		+			++					
small intestine:										
stenosis, tumour, inflammation	++			+						
erosion ulcer	+			++						
ileus, pseudo-obstruction	++				++			+		
disturbed passage	+	+								+
large intestine:										
stenosis, tumour, inflammation	+			++						
dysmotility	+				++			+		
disturbed transport	++	+								
rectum and anus:										
anismus	+*				+*				+*	
anatomical abnormality	++	+		++						
perineal descent syndrome	++									

Table 14: Which investigation is suitable for which disorder?

*Preferably a combination of these techniques.

Conclusion

CONCLUSION

Over the past 20 years, gastroenterology and gastroenterological surgery have changed beyond all recognition. This is primarily because new investigation techniques for objectively examining patients have become available. In addition, new possibilities for treatment have had a tremendous influence on these specialist areas.

Significant progress has been made with regard to motility disorders of the gastrointestinal tract. In this book, we have given an overview of the normal and abnormal movements of the gastrointestinal tract. It is clear that,

compared with the situation 20 years ago, the diagnostic and therapeutic arsenal at the doctor's disposal has expanded dramatically. In cases where previously dysmotility could only have been assumed, it can now be objectively shown. Where previously therapeutic influence on gastrointestinal dysmotility was impossible (or was possible in a highly unselective fashion only, with many undesired side-effects), it is now often possible to effect selective action.

And this is just the beginning. We are convinced that just as much progress will be made over the next 20 years.

Index

Bold page numbers indicate that the entry is also discussed on the following pages.